the little book of aromatherapy

the little book of
aromatherapy

REVISED

Kathi Keville

For Karen
Kathi Keville
HSA 2014

Crossing Press
Berkeley

Published in the United States by Crossing Press, an imprint of the
Crown Publishing Group, a division of Random House, Inc., New York.
www.crownpublishing.com
www.tenspeed.com

Crossing Press and the Crossing Press colophon are registered
trademarks of Random House, Inc.

Library of Congress Cataloging-in-Publication Data

Keville, Kathi.
The little book of aromatherapy / by Kathi Keville.
— Rev., 1st ed.
p. cm.
Rev. ed. of: Pocket guide to aromatherapy. 1996.
Summary: "The updated pocket guide to using essential oil formulas
for enhancing beauty, health, and overall well-being, from a
leading practitioner"—Provided by publisher.
Includes index.
ISBN 978-1-58091-195-5
1. Aromatherapy. I. Keville, Kathi. Pocket guide to aromatherapy. II. Title.
RM666.A68K483 2009
615'.321—dc22
2009014960
ISBN 978-1-58091-195-5

Printed in the United States of America

Design by Katy Brown

10 9 8 7 6 5 4 3 2 1

First Edition

I dedicate this book to everyone who has ever smelled a flower, sniffed the first scent of spring in the air, or walked down the fragrant path of an herb garden. May your lives always be filled with fragrance!

Thank you to all the modern pioneers of aromatherapy who have brought this ancient art to the attention of the world. Thank you especially to aromatherapist Mindy Green, my friend and coauthor of *Aromatherapy: A Complete Guide to the Healing Art*. Her knowledge and inspiration are reflected in this pocket guide.

contents

what is aromatherapy?

Aromatherapy is the use of essential oils—potent aromatic substances extracted from fragrant plants—for physical and emotional healing. Today, herbalists, body workers, cosmetologists, chiropractors, and other holistic healers are discovering how this multifaceted and versatile healing art can enrich their practices. You can use the same principles of aromatherapy as a natural remedy in your home.

Interest in the therapeutic effects of essential oils continues to grow. Essential oils are being pumped into offices, stores, and even some hospitals to make the atmosphere more relaxing. Large corporations are turning to fragrance to keep their workers alert, and more content, on the job. Inhaling certain essential oils has even been shown to lower blood pressure.

There are many approaches to using essential oils. Applied externally, they penetrate through the skin into underlying tissues. They also reach the bloodstream quickly: compounds from lavender oil have been detected in the blood only twenty minutes after the oil was rubbed on the skin. As a result, one can treat a wide range of physical problems with aromatherapy. For example, massaging the appropriate aromatherapy body oil—such as one containing peppermint—on the abdomen will soothe indigestion. Rubbing an aromatic vapor balm on the chest will relieve lung congestion and fight infection, both by being inhaled and drawn deep into the lungs' air passages and by penetrating the skin and reaching the underlying tissue. Aromatherapy cosmetics and skin preparations are also used to counter skin inflammations such as eczema. *Note:* Because essential oils are so concentrated, they must be used carefully. Always dilute them before applying them to your body, and be sure to see a qualified health practitioner in the case of a reaction.

The beauty of aromatherapy is that you can take advantage of both its physical and emotional applications in the same treatment. For example, you can blend a combination of essential oils that will not only stop indigestion but also calm you down and reduce the nervous condition that led to the indigestion, and you can design an aromatherapy body lotion that will not only improve your complexion but also relieve depression.

In the pages that follow, I will describe all of these methods and more, providing plenty of recipes along the way to get you started. I will also touch on the cosmetic applications of aromatherapy in skin- and hair-care products. If I succeed in sparking your interest in aromatherapy, be sure to have a look at the book I wrote with Mindy Green, *Aromatherapy: The Complete Guide to the Healing Art* (also from Crossing Press), which goes into greater detail about using essential oils and making your own aromatherapy products.

questions most frequently asked about aromatherapy

With today's growing emphasis on natural solutions to mind and body issues, people's curiosity about aromatherapy is burgeoning. The following are answers to some of the questions people often ask me.

Is aromatherapy a new science?

Aromatherapy goes back to at least 4000 B.C.E., when Neolithic people made ointments by combining vegetable oils with aromatic plants. Throughout the world, cultures began using aromatic steams, smoke, and water for healing. Around 3000 B.C.E., the uses of odoriferous herbs were recorded on papyrus by the Egyptians and on clay tablets in Mesopotamia and Babylonia. By 1700 B.C.E., trade routes had been established throughout the Middle East, in part to permit traffic in solid aromatic unguents; myrrh and frankincense for incense, perfume, and medicine; and aromatic spices for food. Eventually these routes extended into India, China, and Europe.

Essential oils were probably being distilled in Europe, China, and Japan by about 500 C.E., which led to the development of colognes, perfume, and facial waters. These were not only used to disguise body odor and improve the complexion but also ingested as medicinal tonics.

Appropriately, the birth of modern aromatherapy took place in France, the modern capital of perfume. It was René-Maurice Gattefossé, a French chemist descended from a long line of perfumers, who reunited the arts of perfumery and medicine. He coined the term *aromatherapy* around 1928 following an accident in his family's perfume factory. When a laboratory explosion severely burned his hand, he plunged it into a container of lavender essential oil and was amazed at how quickly the burn healed. Young Gattefossé began to look for an answer. Eventually his writings inspired others to explore aromatherapy. Interest in the new science spread to Europe and finally to the United States. Of course, herbalists were already using aromatic plants in their healing work.

How is aromatherapy connected to herbalism?

Aromatherapy always has been a part of herbalism. In their writings, the ancient Egyptians, Arabs, Greeks, Romans, and European herbalists all referred to the use of fragrance for healing purposes.

If you have ever used herbs, then chances are you have also experienced aromatherapy. Aromatic molecules, called essential oils, occur in any fragrant plant. Whenever you make a tea of, say, peppermint or chamomile, the heat draws essential oils from the plant into the water. You receive the healing benefits of essential oils both as you drink the tea and as you inhale the aroma. It is also possible to extract essential oils directly from herbs into alcohol or warm vegetable oil. (If you have an herb garden or other good supply of fragrant herbs, you may want to experiment.)

Aromatherapy differs from herbalism because it employs only *fragrant* herbs. I like to think of it as one branch of herbalism—one that uses fragrant plants exclusively. Although familiar nonfragrant herbs such as comfrey or goldenseal are not used in aromatherapy, many common medicinal herbs, such as elecampane, angelica, and myrrh, are used. There are other fragrant plants that are not typically used by herbalists but do produce therapeutic essential oils, such as ylang-ylang and vanilla. Because herbs often contain several different types of medicinal compounds besides essential oils, herb books describing a fragrant herb's properties may not always be referring to the properties in the essential oil.

What are essential oils?

Essential oils consist of tiny aromatic molecules that are released from a plant when crushed, rubbed, or heated (as on a hot summer day). This is what makes an herb garden smell so fragrant. Each type of essential oil is composed of many different aromatic molecules—more than thirty thousand have been identified and named, and it is common for a single essential oil to contain one hundred different aromatic molecules.

It's the vast number of possible combinations of these molecules that produces so many unique plant fragrances. As you sniff your way through a selection of essential oils, you'll notice that some plants smell identical or similar. That's because the same fragrant molecules can occur in more than one plant, even when the plants in question are unrelated. This is true of plants that produce a lemonlike aroma; they include lemon itself, lemon verbena, melissa (lemon balm), lemon thyme, lemon eucalyptus, citronella, and palmarosa. Even though all of these plants and their corresponding essential oils smell similar, each one possesses a slightly different combination of aromatic molecules and carries its own distinctive olfactory shading.

In a few cases, a plant's essential oil is composed chiefly of one type of molecule. For example, sandalwood may contain up to 90 percent santalol, and clove bud has between 70 percent and 80 percent eugenol.

Why do plants produce essential oils?

At first, botanists were not sure why plants contain essential oils, which they viewed as mere by-products of plant metabolism. They were at a loss to explain why some plants produce essential oils and others do not, or why the fragrances vary so much from one plant to another.

Although there is still much to learn about why plants are fragrant, modern botanical research now understands that even though plants discard essential oils as waste products, the oils do serve important functions. Many essential oils are highly antiseptic, preventing the growth of bacteria, mold, and fungus on a plant. Fragrances can attract insects that help to fertilize their flowers. They also protect plants by repelling certain insects as well as other predators. Many essential oils contain substances called *terpenes*, which help to waterproof the plant and protect it from rain. (The presence of terpenes in an essential oil also makes it difficult to mix it with water.)

How are essential oils obtained from plants?

The pure essential oils available at the local herb shop are usually extracted from plants through a process called *steam distillation*. Freshly picked plants are suspended over boiling water, and the steam draws the oils out of the plant. The next step is to rapidly cool the steam back into water. During this process, the essential oil separates from the water.

There are several other ways to produce essential oils. One method squeezes, or presses, essential oils from the plant. Another old method, rarely used today, is *enfleurage*, which extracts the oils into sheets of warm fat. Although various solvents may be used to extract essential oils, aromatherapists worry about the possibility of slight traces of the solvent contaminating the oils.

New methods of obtaining essential oils are currently being developed and introduced. One of the most interesting processes (albeit an expensive one) extracts the oil with carbon dioxide and no heat. The resulting essential oils have an odor much like that of the original plant.

Can I make my own essential oils?

You can indeed make essential oils at home—but don't expect to produce much! It isn't unusual to obtain only a small vial of essential oil from a wheelbarrow full of plants. The process is simple, although even a small commercial steam distiller costs several hundred dollars. You can also have a steam distiller custom-built by someone who does laboratory-glass blowing. Check the yellow pages for a chemistry supply house.

There is an inexpensive way to rig up a steam distiller in your kitchen, although you probably won't end up with essential oil.

Instead, you will obtain aromatic waters, also called *hydrosol*—and you may even produce a few drops of oil if you distill plants that yield a lot of oil, such as eucalyptus, rosemary, and peppermint. Whether you purchase a distiller or rig one up at home, you will need to have a large supply of plants. Fresh plants release oil better than dried plants, because plants lose quite a bit of essential oil when they are dried. However, if you don't have your own herb garden, you can still produce essential oils and hydrosols from dried plants.

Why are some essential oils so much more expensive than others?

The broad price range of essential oils—they can vary from $3 to $1,000 per ounce—reflects the range of difficulty involved in cultivating, collecting, producing, and storing different types. It is no wonder that Bulgarian rose oil sells for over $800 an ounce—it took about six hundred pounds of rose petals to produce that ounce! Plus, rose bushes must be carefully cultivated, pruned, and hand-harvested. On the other hand, plants such as eucalyptus and rosemary are easy to grow and yield a comparatively large amount of essential oil, placing them among the least expensive oils.

How does fragrance affect emotions?

When your olfactory sensors detect a particular aroma, this information is sent to areas of the brain that influence memory, learning, emotions, hormone balance, and basic survival mechanisms. Exactly how the brain processes this data is not completely understood, but we do know that certain fragrances act on the brain's primitive limbic system, also known as the *smell brain*.

Researchers studying aromachology—the science of medicinal aromas—have discovered that exposure to aromatic substances results in an alteration of brain waves. They suspect that aromas work on the brain in other ways. The fragrance research company International Fragrance and Flavor has tested over two thousand subjects to better understand how certain scents relieve pain, call up deep-seated memories, and affect personality, behavior, and sleep patterns.

It is no surprise that some psychologists incorporate aromatherapy into their practices. In France in the 1960s, psychologist Jean Valnet used vanilla to help his patients unlock childhood memories. Nowadays, psychologists use aromatherapy to help patients overcome anxiety and other emotional problems through association. They first create a state of relaxation, often through pleasant music, then introduce a scent. After several exposures to relaxation with the same scent, the patient begins to associate it with a tranquil state. The patients then carry that scent with them, and whenever they encounter a situation that makes them tense, nervous, or anxious, they open the bottle, sniff, and relax. Several large Tokyo corporations have followed the advice of staff psychologists and circulate lemon, peppermint, and cypress through their air-conditioning systems to keep workers attentive—and reduce the urge to smoke. Aroma is also used to assist truck drivers, railroad engineers, air traffic controllers, and others whose jobs require that they remain alert.

Why are so many cosmetologists working with aromatherapy?

Many large cosmetics firms—including Aveda, Revlon, Redken, Avon, Charles of the Ritz, and Japan's Shiseido—have discovered that aromatherapy offers a complete health and beauty package for both skin and hair care. Actually, this is nothing new. Fragrant herbs have long been used to clear complexions and make hair silky. Certain essential oils stimulate oil production in dry skin and hair. Others slow down overactive oil glands. Many of the oils also soothe and heal irritated skin. There are a few companies that add essential oils and botanical derivatives only to cash in on the current popularity of anything natural; these companies don't always choose the most appropriate ingredients. Be sure to read the labels carefully when choosing skin-care products. Or you can make your own aromatherapy products for a fraction of what you would pay at the store.

Can I learn to like scents that bother me at first?

Not everyone likes the same fragrances. I know people who have felt uncomfortable around someone else who wears the same cologne or perfume as another person with whom they have had problems. One man in my class hated the smell of lavender because the funeral parlor in his hometown used it. Many people in his family died when he was young; as a result, he came to associate lavender with grief. No matter how many books say that lavender is relaxing and promotes smiling, if you associate that fragrance with a bad memory, you may never learn to enjoy it. It takes time to change a negative reaction to a fragrance, and it's not always possible. If this is the case, don't despair—aromatherapy offers so many different and appealing fragrances, you can afford to let one go.

*Nature imitates all things
in flowers. They are at
once the most beautiful
and the ugliest objects, the
most fragrant and the most
offensive to the nostrils.*

—THOREAU

creating formulas: getting started

Making and using aromatherapy products for healing or skin care is not difficult. Some basic information about essential oils and a few safety tips are all you need to conduct your first experiments. Start by making simple remedies and a few essential oils. As you become more familiar with the fragrances and properties of the different oils, the process will become easier and easier. Follow the suggestions in the next five chapters and take inspiration from the descriptions of individual oils in the Materia Medica section at the back of the book. Use your nose as your guide, and don't be afraid to experiment. Be sure to take careful notes so that you can duplicate an effective combination—or avoid repeating one that didn't work out. Always keep in mind that the most effective aromatherapy preparations have a subtle fragrance.

safety

Aromatherapy is an excellent resource for mind/body health, but only when used properly. The following are some tips about the proper use of essential oils, which are very concentrated and therefore must be used carefully. I estimate that just one or two drops of essential oil is roughly equivalent to the amount of essential oil in a regular cup of tea. That means that each drop is very potent, making it easy to overdose with essential oils.

❋ Always dilute essential oils before applying them to your body. They are so concentrated that an overdose can occur easily, even with relatively "safe" oils. Overdoses tax and can harm the liver and kidneys. These organs of elimination are responsible for clearing the body of toxins, including an overabundance of essential oils.

❋ If you accidentally spill essential oil on yourself, immediately wipe it off and use any type of alcohol, if available, to remove the residue. It's also a good idea to take herbs that are beneficial to the liver and kidneys, such as burdock, milk thistle, and dandelion. Since I work with essential oils, I keep an extract of these herbs on hand.

❋ Overexposure to essential oils, either through the skin or by nose, can result in nausea, headache, skin irritation, emotional unease, or a "spaced out" feeling. Getting some fresh air and having adequate ventilation (an air filter if necessary) will help you to avoid or overcome these symptoms.

❋ Try to limit your use of essential oils to a few drops a day. That includes the oils in all products, such as mouthwash that contains essential oils.

❋ If you want to use an essential oil internally, your best bet is to ingest the herb from which it is derived as a tea, capsule, or tincture instead of the essential oil, which can burn the inside of your mouth and is quickly absorbed into the blood system.

❋ Many essential oils can burn or irritate skin, so always dilute them before use. Keep all essential oils away from your eyes. If you experience skin irritation from essential oils, or you accidentally get some in your eyes, flush with straight vegetable oil—not water, which will not dilute the oils.

❋ Use essential oils cautiously with anyone who is elderly or convalescing, and carefully—or not at all—with people who have serious liver or kidney problems. These organs are responsible for clearing the body of essential oils, so this will increase their workload. Insufficient clearing of the oils can result in a high concentration and overdose.

❋ A few people have allergies or sensitivities to essential oils. If there is any chance of this, run a patch test, mixing one drop of the suspect essential oil in one-quarter teaspoon of vegetable oil and placing a drop of the mixture in the crook of the arm. Wait twelve hours to see if a reaction occurs. If someone has a known allergy to a certain plant, the person may or may not be allergic to its essential oil, but it is better to avoid its use. When a person is allergic to nuts, don't use almond or other nut oils as a carrier oil.

❋ If you are using essential oils over several months, vary the ones you use to avoid overexposure to any one oil.

❋ Photosensitizing oils react on the skin of a few individuals. This can produce an uneven pigmentation on the skin of a few people, so use these carefully—and never in a suntan lotion. The most notorious is bergamot, which contains bergaptene, a powerful photosensitizer.

❋ Toxic oils are not included in the Materia Medica (page 121) because they are too toxic for general use. Semitoxic oils should be used very cautiously. Never use either category for the elderly, children, or pregnant women.

Potential Skin Irritants

Bay rum

Black pepper

Citronella

Thuja

Birch

Cinnamon

Clove

Thyme (except linalol type)

Photosensitizing Essential Oils

Angelica

Bergamot

Orange

Slightly Photosensitizing Essential Oils

Cumin

Lemon

Lime

Potentially Toxic Essential Oils

Mugwort (*Artemesia vulgaris*)

Pennyroyal (*Mentha pelugium*)

Sassafras (*Sassafras albidum*)

Savory (*Satureja hortensis*)

Tansy (*Tanacetum anuum*)

Thuja (*Thuja occidentalis*)

Wormwood (*Artemisia arborescens*)

Bitter almond (*Prunus amygdalus*, var. *amara*)
Hyssop (*Hyssopus officinalis*)
Oregano (*Origanum vulgare*)

equipment and supplies

Unless you plan to extract your own essential oils, you will need little equipment to make aromatherapy preparations at home. Your kitchen probably contains almost everything you need. Vegetable oils (such as almond, apricot, grape seed, and coconut) and jojoba wax are available in most natural-food stores.

The glass droppers you need to measure out small amounts of the essential oils and transfer them from one bottle to the next are sold in drug stores and in some natural-food stores. A dropper is usually accurate enough, although be aware that the size of a drop will vary slightly depending on the size of the dropper opening, the temperature, and the thickness (viscosity) of the essential oil. Although it is important not to contaminate your essential oils by moving the dropper directly from one vial of oil to the next, you don't need to have a separate dropper for each of the oils. Simply rinse the oily dropper in a small bottle of alcohol (such as vodka or rubbing alcohol) and wait a few minutes for the alcohol to completely evaporate before putting the dropper into another bottle.

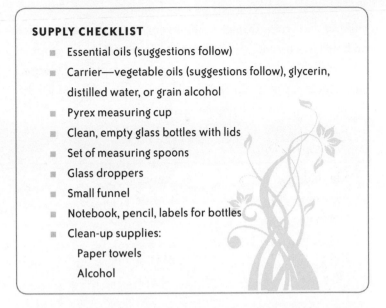

SUPPLY CHECKLIST

- Essential oils (suggestions follow)
- Carrier—vegetable oils (suggestions follow), glycerin, distilled water, or grain alcohol
- Pyrex measuring cup
- Clean, empty glass bottles with lids
- Set of measuring spoons
- Glass droppers
- Small funnel
- Notebook, pencil, labels for bottles
- Clean-up supplies:
    Paper towels
    Alcohol

Besides kitchen equipment, you will need a few basic essential oils. These are sold at many natural-food stores and herb stores, as well as through mail-order catalogs (see Resources, page 155).

Carrier Oils

To make the simplest aromatherapy product, put a few drops of essential oils into a carrier oil, and you're done! The resulting oil can be used as body, massage, or bath oil. A typical aromatherapy application adds ten to twelve drops essential oil per ounce of a carrier, such as almond oil. This is a 2-percent dilution. Half that amount of essential oil (a 1-percent solution) is better for children, pregnant women, and anyone in weak health. When making large batches, you will find it easier to measure essential oils by the teaspoon, rather than drop by drop! See Dilutions and Doses, page 151, for the number of drops you need for different types of aromatherapy preparations.

Popular Carrier Oils

Almond	Apricot
Avocado	Castor
Coconut	Grape Seed
Hazelnut	Jojoba
Kukui	Macadamia
Olive	Sesame

incorporating herbs into aromatherapy

When combined together, herbs and essential oils have a greater capacity for healing than one has by itself. You can prepare salves, lotions, and creams by adding essential oils. Oils made by soaking herbs in vegetable oil, called *infused oils*, may be used as the carrier oil in place of plain vegetable oil to make the medicines more potent. Examples are arnica, calendula, and St. John's wort oils, which all help heal injured skin. You can purchase infused oils or make your own.

tips for creating custom formulas

The many choices that go into the creation of a blend may seem intimidating at first, but they also add to the excitement. Remember to keep records of how you make your preparations; include ingredients, proportions, processing procedures, and comments. Label your finished products with the ingredients, date, and any special instructions. When combining essential oils in a therapeutic blend, it is easiest for a beginner to use no more than three oils at a time. That way you will avoid unpredictable results due to the complex chemistries involved.

ESSENTIAL OIL STARTER KIT	
Oil	*For relief of*
Chamomile	indigestion, stress, allergies, rashes, muscle cramps, inflammation, anxiety, anger, and depression
Geranium	imbalance of mind and body
Lavender	infection, inflammation, insomnia, pain, depression, and anxiety
Lemon (or other citrus)	infections, depression, parasites
Peppermint	indigestion, sinus congestion, itching, panic, fatigue
Rosemary	pain, congestion, grief; poor circulation and memory
Tea tree	infection, fatigue

Don't worry—you can create an effective remedy with just one or two oils.

I like to create an aromatherapy product by first deciding the medicinal use, both physically and emotionally. After that, I turn my attention to making it smell fantastic by adjusting the proportions and making substitutions when necessary. Finally, I measure my drops. While you're blending, be aware that your nose will quickly become accustomed to the scent and you will no longer be able to accurately perceive the fragrance of the blend you are making. I suggest walking away, then waiting at least fifteen minutes before coming back to your blend with a fresh nose. If you have the luxury of being able to create your blend over several days, take it slow, giving yourself time to make subtle adjustments. You'll notice that blends change as the oils blend together over a few weeks.

With experience, you'll be able to imagine how the blend will smell while you're designing the formula and then predict the direction it will take as the individual oils blend together. Practice is your best instructor when you're learning how to make aromatherapy blends.

When you start blending essential oils, you may wish to take a few hints from professional perfumers, who consider the *top notes*, *middle notes*, and *low notes*. These terms define how heavy or light the scent appears. A fragrance that is light and airy, like lavender, contains many top notes. Those that are heavy and lingering—patchouli and vetiver, for example—are predominantly low notes. The middle notes, found in an herb like marjoram, lie in between. Perfume smells most intriguing and attractive when it contains all three notes. When you are learning how to blend oils, avoid those that smell very pungent or sharp. For example, a blend of eucalyptus, tea tree, and rosemary smells sharp and medicinal.

Essential oils vary in odor intensity, so some oils should be added to your blends in smaller amounts than other, less intensely fragrant oils. As you work with them, you'll notice oils with a high odor intensity—such as chamomile, patchouli, cinnamon, ylang-ylang, and clary sage—just by smelling them. Usually, using one drop per ounce of these intense oils is sufficient. Also, avoid using too many of them in the same formula until you have enough blending experience to keep them from overpowering the combination.

If all this talk about notes and intensity is making you nervous, here are a few shortcuts for beginning aromatherapists.

HOMEMADE HERBAL OIL

Oils made by steeping herbs in vegetable oil are called *infusions*. They can be used in aromatherapy preparation in place of plain carrier oils. To prepare, place finely chopped dried herbs in a wide-mouth glass jar and add just enough vegetable oil to completely cover the herbs. Put the jar in a warm place— in a sunny window, a crock pot set very low, or by a heater—for two to three days with constant heat, three to seven days if the temperature fluctuates. The oil will take on the color and scent of the herbs. Strain through a strainer or cheesecloth, bottle, and store in a cool place.

Start with an essential oil that has a fairly complex chemistry and already smells like a blend. One example is geranium, which contains hints of several different botanicals—rose, pine, cedarwood, and citrus. You can then expand your formula by adding small amounts of these oils, one at a time. Your choices depend on the direction in which you want to move the scent of the blend.

Another interesting way to expand a blend is to choose oils that smell similar to each other. This performs a delightful trick on the nose when the oils begin to play off one another, making your blend seem more complicated and mysterious. Try combining mints such as peppermint and spearmint, citrus such as lemon and bergamot, or spice scents like cinnamon and ginger. Every choice you make will take your blend in a new and interesting direction.

regarding quality

To make a quality product, you will need to start with quality essential oils. Factors determining quality include purity, growing conditions, differences among species, extraction techniques, and proper storage. You may not always need the highest grade of essential oil, but know what you are buying and make sure it is a pure oil that has not been diluted with a cheaper oil or a solvent to extend it. The best advice for judging quality is to train your nose. Your sense of smell will become keener as you continue to work with good-quality essential oils. Once you are familiar with pure, undiluted essential oils made from plants, poor-quality and synthetic oils will never smell the same. An excellent way to train your nose is to attend an aromatherapy seminar. I always warn my students that the seminar will make their sense of smell so discerning, it will spoil them for life.

Another way to educate your nose is to go into a store that offers essential oils from several companies and see if you can smell the difference. Enter the store armed with a little knowledge, and don't be shy about asking questions so you can tell whether the staff person is knowledgeable about essential oils. I've encountered store clerks who think that any product marked "essential oil" is natural. When buying essential oils, keep in mind that some of the best aromatherapy companies are run by aromatherapists, who stake their reputations on supplying good essential oils.

Purity

Purity is of concern to anyone purchasing essential oils. Rare and expensive oils are the most likely candidates for adulteration. This can be done by diluting or "extending" them with vegetable oil, alcohol, or another solvent. You can determine whether essential oil has been diluted with vegetable oil by placing a small drop on a piece of paper or cloth. Because they evaporate so easily, most essential oils leave no stain. The exceptions are dark oils, such as patchouli, benzoin, and German chamomile (verses Roman or other types of chamomile), and thick oils, like sandalwood. Oils extended by adding alcohol can be detected by a slight "boozy" odor. It is more difficult to tell when essential oil is diluted with an odorless, non-oily solvent, which is especially problematic because solvents can be absorbed through the skin and inhaled through the lungs. You'll notice that diluted essential oils smell weaker than the pure version.

Oils that have been adulterated with similar but less expensive oils smell altered. Unfortunately, it can be difficult for an untrained nose to tell the difference between expensive pure essential oil of lemon verbena or melissa and those same oils mixed with the cheaper lemongrass or citronella. In fact, these two oils are so often adulterated that you may never have smelled the real thing. An essential oil that is cut with another oil will not have the same properties.

Essential Oil Grades

Many essential oils are available in different grades that reflect where the oil came from and the plants' growing conditions. A good example is lavender, available in a number of different grades and also as different species and subspecies. This is why you will probably encounter many different lavenders. When essential oils smell different from each other, it doesn't necessarily indicate that one is inferior, but the higher-grade essential oils generally carry more of a bouquet, a fuller-bodied fragrance. When there are variations between oils of comparable quality, personal preference can be your guide. Of course, poorer-quality oils can cost more in the long run. A friend who makes facial creams had to use four times as much essential oil to achieve the same results after she switched to an inferior grade.

Avoid Synthetic Oils

As I mentioned earlier, when I pass around high-quality essential oils in my aromatherapy seminars, I warn the students that once you have smelled the real thing, it is difficult to accept using anything less. Synthetics, usually made with petroleum-based chemicals, are an attempt to duplicate natural scents; in my opinion, they never come close. They also are potentially harmful, as their tiny molecules penetrate the skin and enter the bloodstream.

Sad to say, synthetic fragrances permeate our lives. Many body-care products sold in natural-food stores contain them. Most fruits and flowers oils do not naturally produce essential oils, so when you see "essential oil" of carnation, lily of the valley, strawberry, or gardenia, you can be sure these are synthetics. When people say that they react adversely or are allergic to fragrances, I always suspect that they have encountered only synthetics.

proper storage

Once you've gone to the trouble of locating and purchasing quality essential oils, you will want to keep them that way. Store them in dark glass vials with tight lids in a cool place out of direct sunlight. Properly stored, most essential oils will keep for years.

Citrus oils, such as orange and lemon, are the most vulnerable to oxidation and spoilage, but even they can last a couple of years if refrigerated. A few essential oils—such as patchouli, clary sage, benzoin, vetiver, and sandalwood—actually improve with age. (I have thirty-year-old patchouli that smells so rich and vanilla-like, people have trouble identifying the fragrance—even those who say that they hate the smell of patchouli.)

It is important to always keep pure essential oils in glass containers; they will eventually eat away plastic, contaminating the oil. For the same reason, I prefer to also store most diluted aromatherapy products in glass, unless I'm traveling or need a squeeze bottle to give a massage. In that case, I use containers made of a durable, stiff plastic.

When I pick or crush in my
hand a twig of bay, or brush
against a bush of rosemary, or
tread upon a tuft of thyme, or
pass through incense-laden cistus,
I feel that here is all that is best
and purest and most refined, and
nearest to poetry in the range
of faculty of the sense of smell.

—GERTRUDE JEKYLL

aromatherapy and emotional health

How aroma affects the mind is not completely understood, although we do know that when you smell anything, information is sent to the specific areas of the brain that influence memory, learning, emotions, hormone balance, and even basic survival mechanisms such as the fight-or-flight response (an adrenal function). There are psychologists who use fragrances to encourage communication among people. Researchers are finding that pleasant smells make people more willing to negotiate, cooperate, and compromise with others. If you are a health-care practitioner, one subtle way to use aromatherapy with patients is to dab a small amount of an appropriate essential oil on the back of your hand. You can also scent the room using the techniques that have already been suggested (in a diffuser, potpourri cooker, or pan of simmering water, or on a light-bulb ring).

The formulas in this section dilute essential oils with vegetable oil so they can be used as body, massage, or bath oils. Use your choice of vegetable oil, such as grape seed, almond, sesame, or olive oil. (Remember that essential oils should be diluted in something, such as vegetable oil, before being used on the skin.) Simply rub the blend onto the skin for either massage or body oil. A nice time to rub body oil on is after taking a shower. For bath oil, add 1 to 2 teaspoons of the blend to your bath. (See page 75 for more on creating and using aromatherapy bath oils, and Carrier Oils, page 23, for a list of appropriate vegetable oils for body, bath, and massage oils.) If you are working with someone in a health-care situation and do not want to apply the oil to them directly, you can rub the body oil on the inside of your arm. The scent will lightly float around you as you care for the individual and have a positive emotional impact on you both.

*Flowers leave some
of their fragrance in the
hand that bestows them.*

—CHINESE PROVERB

depression

Certain fragrances affect brain waves in a fashion similar to antidepressant drugs, according to research by the Olfaction Research Group at Warwick University in England. At his Istituto di Richerche sui Derivati Vegetali clinic in Milan, Italy, psychologist Dr. Paolo Rovesti successfully lifted many patients out of depression in the 1970s and 1980s with the citrus scents

Antidepressant Essential Oils

Angelica	Bergamot
Cedarwood	Chamomile
Citruses	Clary sage
Cypress	Geranium
Grapefruit	Helichrysum
Jasmine	Lavender
Lemon verbena	Marjoram
Melissa	Neroli
Patchouli	Pine
Petitgrain	Rose
Sandalwood	Vetiver
Ylang-ylang	

of orange, bergamot, lemon, and lemon verbena. Sixteenth-century herbalist John Gerard said that melissa "gladdens the heart" and that clary sage counters depression, paranoia, mental fatigue, and nervous disorders. One of my favorite citrus antidepressants is the elegant-scented neroli (orange blossom) essential oil.

ANTIDEPRESSANT FORMULA

Try this formula whenever you are feeling down or have just had a bad day and need a lift. You can sniff it throughout the day, but my favorite way to counter depression with aromatherapy is with an aromatic bath. It will wash away the cares of the world. If you do happen to be on antidepressant drugs, feel free to use aromatherapy; it will not interfere.

- **6 drops bergamot**
- **3 drops petitgrain**
- **3 drops rose geranium**
- **1 drop neroli (expensive, so it's optional)**
- **2 ounces vegetable oil**

Combine the essential oils with the vegetable oil. Massage into skin as body oil, use as massage oil, or add 2 teaspoons to a bath.

anxiety

Aromatherapists use several fragrances to help overcome feelings of anxiety, loneliness, and rejection. I find the same oils are useful for anyone undergoing a major life transition.

Essential Oils to Relieve Anxiety

Basil	Bergamot
Cardamom	Chamomile
Cypress	Fennel
Frankincense	Geranium
Jasmine	Juniper
Lavender	Marjoram
Melissa	Myrrh
Neroli	Orange
Peppermint	Petitgrain
Pine	Rose
Vanilla	

ANTIANXIETY FORMULA

Life is full of anxiety-creating situations. This blend will calm your mind and help you to refocus. You can program your mind to relax before going out into any setting that causes you anxiety. Find a calming environment where you can listen to music that you find relaxing while smelling this blend. Whenever you inhale the same aroma, you'll associate it with relaxation and feel less anxious. If you want to carry this scent around with you, smelling salts are a convenient way to do so. Make them by combining the essential oils listed below with a tablespoon of rock salt instead of the vegetable oil. (Salt absorbs the oils and makes the scent last longer than it would as pure oil carried around in a vial.) Let the scents blend in a lidded glass jar for a day, then pour a few pieces of the now-scented salt into a well-sealed vial to keep in your purse or pocket. Whenever you feel the need, open the vial and take a sniff.

6 drops lavender
3 drops orange
1 drop marjoram
1 drop cedarwood
2 ounces vegetable oil

Combine the essential oils with the vegetable oil. Massage into skin as body oil, use as massage oil, or add 2 teaspoons to a bath.

fatigue

A Japanese manufacturer has designed an alarm clock that awaken sleepers by spraying out the scents of eucalyptus and pine. At several large Tokyo companies, lemon, cypress, and peppermint circulate through the air-conditioning systems throughout the workday to keep employees alert. The spicy aromas of clove, basil, black pepper, cinnamon, and, to a lesser degree, patchouli and lemongrass, are known to reduce drowsiness, irritability, and headaches. They have been found to prevent the sharp drop in attention typical after thirty minutes of work, but they don't over-amp the adrenal glands like caffeine. In the early 1920s, Italian doctor-researchers Giovanni Gatti and Renato Cayola used clove, cinnamon, lemon, ylang-ylang, cardamom, fennel, and angelica to make patients feel more alert and responsive.

Stimulating Essential Oils

Angelica	Basil
Black pepper	Cardamom
Cinnamon	Clove
Cypress	Eucalyptus
Lemon	Peppermint

STIMULANT FORMULA

We all encounter times when we need to perk up and be more alert. A few sniffs of this blend should help anyone who needs to wake up. The good news is that it won't interfere with sleep, even as soon as an hour or so after use. If you want help staying alert while driving or typing, drop the following essential oils (without the vegetable oil) onto a small piece of cardboard to hang from your car's mirror or keep by the computer. Feel free to decorate the cardboard to give it that personal touch!

7 drops lemon
2 drops eucalyptus
2 drops peppermint
1 drop cinnamon
2 ounces vegetable oil

Combine the essential oils with the vegetable oil. Dab onto skin for an energizing uplift. You can also use it as a stimulating body oil, making sure to keep it away from the eyes and sensitive areas, as it contains some hot oils.

poor memory

Researchers have learned that mental recall improves dramati-
cally when a past event is associated with smell. That's why a
whiff of a perfume or other fragrance can send you back in time,
evoking long-forgotten images and feelings. Next to my computer I keep a sprig of rosemary, whose ability to increase memory, concentration, and even creativity is legendary. Modern
Japanese research confirms that rosemary is a brain stimulant.

Memory-Stimulating Essential Oils

Anise	Bay laurel
Cardamom	Clove
Fennel	Lavender
Lemon	Lemon verbena
Melissa	Peppermint
Rosemary	Thyme

MEMORY FORMULA

Dab some of this body oil onto your temples or elsewhere while studying or working for a memory boost. You'll thank yourself at that test or meeting later!

5 drops lavender
4 drops lemon
3 drops rosemary
1 drop cinnamon
2 ounces vegetable oil

Combine the essential oils with the vegetable oil. Massage into skin as body oil, use as massage oil, or add a couple of teaspoons to a bath.

grief

In the sixteenth century, herbalist John Gerard wrote that basil "taketh away sorrowfulness . . . and maketh a man merry and glad" and suggested a whiff of marjoram "for those given to much sighing" due to grief, loneliness, or rejection. Ancient Egyptians, Greeks, and Romans sniffed marjoram to strengthen emotions. The Greeks used cypress and hyssop to comfort mourners; several ancient cultures burned sandalwood at death ceremonies to accomplish the same purpose. In Europe, the scents of sage, clary sage, and rosemary were used to overcome grief. Modern-day aromatherapists recommend these same essential oils during any difficult transition in one's life, such as a job change or the end of a romantic relationship. A good companion oil is gentle, relaxing lavender, which is used traditionally to comfort the sick or anyone feeling emotionally upset.

Essential Oils to Ease Grief

Cypress	Fir
Frankincense	Juniper
Marjoram	Rose
Rosemary	Sage

GRIEF-RESOLVING FORMULA

Grief and sadness are natural parts of life. Aroma has long been used to help an individual who is experiencing these emotions feel better. A traditional way to use grief-resolving formulas was to place a drop or two of the following blend (without the vegetable oil) on a hanky. If overcome with emotion, the individual could politely bring the scented hanky up to the face and inhale deeply. If you don't feel like reviving the hanky tradition, add scent to facial tissues. To do so, place 11 drops of the essential oil blend on the top of a cardboard box of tissues. Enclose the box in a sealed, plastic bag and leave it for about five days to allow the scent to disperse, then remove it. The scent will be light, but noticeable on all the tissues.

- **4 drops marjoram**
- **3 drops melissa or lemon**
- **2 drops clary sage**
- **2 drops cypress or rosemary**
- **2 ounces vegetable oil**

Combine the essential oils with the vegetable oil. Massage into skin as body oil, use as massage oil, or add 2 teaspoons to a soothing bath.

insomnia

Lack of sleep is a problem for millions of Americans, often leading to tiredness, poor concentration, agitation, depression, dizziness, and headaches. The scents of the following essential oils go right to the brain to cause relaxation and lull you to sleep.

Essential Oils for Insomnia

Anise	Bergamot
Chamomile	Cypress
Fennel	Frankincense
Geranium	Jasmine
Lavender	Lemon
Lemon verbena	Marjoram
Melissa (lemon balm)	Myrrh
Neroli (orange blossom)	Petitgrain
Rose	Sage
Sandalwood	Ylang-ylang

INSOMNIA FORMULA

An excellent way to encourage sleep is to take a small pillow (avoid silk, which can stain) and dab the following essential oil blend (without the vegetable oil) on it. Put the pillow in a sealed plastic bag for at least two days so the scent can permeate it, then keep it on your bed ready to grab and sniff whenever insomnia lurks. I travel with my aromatherapy pillow and find it is a familiar sleep aid when I'm away from home. If you're feeling creative, sew two squares of fabric together on three sides to make a pouch, then fill it with herbs. Sprinkle the essential oils on the herbs before sewing the fourth side closed, and you'll have a homemade aromatherapy sleep pillow.

- **6 drops bergamot**
- **3 drops chamomile**
- **3 drops geranium**
- **1 drop frankincense**
- **1 drop rose**
- **2 ounces vegetable oil**

Combine the essential oils with the vegetable oil. Massage into skin as body oil, use as massage oil, or add 1 to 2 teaspoons to an evening bath.

stress and nervousness

Fragrance can lower a too-rapid pulse and breathing rate. International Flavors and Fragrance (IFF) researchers have patented a blend of neroli, valerian, and nutmeg to ease stress in the workplace. When past IFF researcher Henry G. Walter, Jr., placed people in a room scented with lavender, bergamot, marjoram, sandalwood, lemon, or chamomile, they tended to mingle more and were less competitive. According to the subjects' brain-

Essential Oils to Reduce Stress

Angelica	Anise
Basil	Benzoin
Bergamot	Cardamom
Cedarwood	Chamomile
Cinnamon	Clary sage
Clove	Eucalyptus
Fennel	Frankincense
Helichrysum	Jasmine
Juniper	Lavender
Lemon	Lemon verbena
Marjoram	Melissa
Myrrh	Neroli
Orange	Petitgrain
Rose	Sandalwood
Valerian	Vanilla
Ylang-ylang	

wave reactions, all of these scents produced a relaxing effect. In the twentieth century, Italian doctors and researchers Giovanni Gatti and Renato Cayola found that the most sedating oils were neroli, petitgrain, chamomile, valerian, and a low-grade myrrh called opopanax. Aromatherapists also classify ylang-ylang among the most potent aromatherapy relaxants.

SEDATIVE FORMULA

Use this formula at the office, at home when the kids are bouncing off the walls, or whenever life seems overwhelming. It will help reduce any type of emotional stress. I like to turn this formula into an aromatherapy spray by adding the essential oil blend (without the vegetable oil) to 1 ounce of distilled water. Be sure to shake the bottle to redistribute the oils just before every use. You can keep a spray bottle at work, in the car, and at home. Use it like an air freshener to spray the immediate environment—or even spray it directly on yourself. Just be sure to close your eyes!

> **4 drops lavender**
> **2 drops sandalwood or cedarwood**
> **2 drops bergamot**
> **2 drops chamomile**
> **1 drop ylang-ylang**
> **2 drops petitgrain**
> **2 ounces vegetable oil**

Combine the essential oils with the vegetable oil. Massage into skin as body oil, use as massage oil, or add 2 to 3 teaspoons to a calming bath.

aphrodisiacs

Research tells us that many of the fragrances known traditionally as aphrodisiacs both stimulate and relax brain waves. Need to relax your partner? Ylang-ylang, rose, patchouli, sandalwood, jasmine, and cinnamon are stimulating aphrodisiacs that also relieve stress.

Aphrodisiac Oils

Cinnamon	Jasmine
Patchouli	Rose
Sandalwood	Vanilla
Ylang-ylang	

APHRODISIAC FORMULA

Want a little spark in your love life? This should do the trick. This is a great blend to use like a perfume. Add the essential oil blend (without the vegetable oil) to $^1/_2$ ounce of brandy (yes, that's right, brandy!) that is at least 100 proof. Dab it on as perfume behind your ears and on your wrists, or be creative! This version of a natural perfume will not last very long, but it smells exquisite while it does.

- **8 drops jasmine**
- **8 drops vanilla**
- **2 drops ylang-ylang**
- **½ drop cinnamon bark**
- **2 ounces vegetable oil**

Combine the essential oils with the vegetable oil. Massage into skin as body oil, use as massage oil, or add 2 teaspoons to a bath.

spiritual scents

Throughout the world, ancient cultures have regarded incense as a mediator between worshipper and deity. Strong aromas with "heavenly" scents were used to aid purification. Prayers were sent into the smoke from the burning incense to communicate between the worlds. A special reverence was given to trees, for they seemed to join earth and sky, representing the mundane with the divine. Rosemary and marjoram represented both birth and death, and were used at weddings and funerals. Lavender is still burned with heavier resins such as myrrh in some Greek Orthodox churches. Sandalwood, frankincense, myrrh, cedarwood (including the famous cedars of Lebanon), juniper, cypress, and camphor were just a few of the ancient holy trees.

Essential Oils to Enhance Spirituality

Cedarwood	Cypress
Frankincense	Juniper
Lavender	Marjoram
Myrrh	Rose
Rosemary	Sandalwood

SPIRITUAL FORMULA

The essential oils in this aromatic formula are drawn from several cultures. An ideal way to use this blend is as anointing oil. These oils have been used by cultures around the world during blessings or to prepare the worshipper for prayer or meditation by placing a drop on the forehead, over the heart, or on the hands.

4 drops sandalwood
4 drops cedarwood
3 drops lavender
1 drop frankincense
1 drop myrrh
1 drop spikenard
1 ounce vegetable oil

Combine the essential oils with the vegetable oil. Massage into skin as body oil, use as massage oil, or add 1 teaspoon to a meditative bath.

aromatherapy
and skin care

The techniques and the essential oils you choose for your over-all skin care should be based on your complexion type. The main types are (1) a mature complexion that is generally dry, (2) oily skin, and (3) a "problem" complexion, associated with conditions such as blackheads and acne. Many people have skin that falls into more than one skin type category, especially on their face. Treat this type of "combination" complexion with a combination of techniques. Although the oils recommended in this chapter are suggested according to how they act on the complexion, keep in mind that they will work on the emotions at the same time.

facial techniques

A facial is one of the kindest things you can give your complexion. The complete treatment includes cleansing, steaming, and exfoliating with a mask, topped off with a facial toner or cream. All of these techniques increase circulation, giving your face a healthful and radiant glow. The entire facial, but especially the skin toners, may also be used for an allover body treatment.

Cleansing

Remove makeup with a water-soluble cleansing cream that won't remove natural skin oils. After removing any makeup, thoroughly cleanse your face. An alternative to soap, which can be harsh because it makes your skin alkaline, is ground oatmeal mixed with enough water to create a cleansing paste. Add a drop of your choice of essential oil that is appropriate for your complexion type (see the following instructions). Gently scrub your face with this mixture, then rinse off. If you have an oily complexion and desire a little more scrubbing action, add cornmeal to the oatmeal. But don't scrub too much, or your skin will be encouraged to produce more oil. Avoid products containing almond husk, which is too abrasive for any skin type. Cleanse oily or problem skin twice a day, dry skin only once a day. Problem skin types can tolerate a neutral pH soap or cleansing gel, but scrubbing and exfoliants only aggravate acne.

FACIAL SCRUB

This scrub will revitalize your skin, leaving you feeling ready to face the day—or night. You can keep a small amount next to your bathroom basin and use it on your face instead of soap.

3 tablespoons oatmeal
1 tablespoon cornmeal (optional)
Water, tea, or hydrosol to moisten

Grind the oats and cornmeal in an electric coffee grinder. Store the powder in a closed container. To use the scrub, moisten one teaspoon with enough water, tea, or hydrosol to make a paste. Apply to a dampened face. Gently scrub and rinse with warm water.

Steaming

Steaming acts as a mini sauna for your face. Besides cleansing and leaving your face looking youthful and vibrant, steaming moisturizes skin and unclogs pores. The heat of the steam increases circulation, which helps cell metabolism. Steaming may be done a few times a week, unless your complexion is extremely dry or delicate. If so, restrict steaming to five minutes every other week. Avoid steaming altogether if you have couperose skin, which easily reddens from small, broken blood vessels just under the skin's surface.

The Facial Mask

A facial mask is a type of exfoliation. It removes dead skin cells from the skin's surface, uncovering young, fresh skin, and stimulates growth of underlying cells. It also draws water from underlying levels to the surface. This temporarily plumps up skin, magically making enlarged pores and wrinkles seem to disappear. As a result, even drying masks can serve as moisturizers and (depending on the ingredients) remineralize the skin. Avoid the chemical exfoliants used in some beauty salons.

Instead, turn to astringent masks of oats, cream of wheat, and clay to exfoliate skin. Gentler masks made with honey, avocado, egg whites, and fresh fruits such as papaya and yogurt are preferred for a delicate or dry complexion. Any of these ingredients can be put together into different combinations. Adding a teaspoon of ground, dried, skin-healing herbs will increase the exfoliation power. Use herbs such as rosemary, or rose petals, for a gentler action.

EXFOLIATING MASK

Your face will thank you if you can take time to do this natural mask once a week.

> **1 tablespoon finely ground oats, or clay powder**
> **1 teaspoon honey, slightly heated**
> **1–2 teaspoons aloe vera juice (or herb tea)**
> **1 drop lavender**

Mash oats or clay with the honey and aloe to form a thin paste. Stir in the essential oil. Apply to the face in an even layer, avoiding sensitive areas around eyes and mouth. Leave on for 5 to 30 minutes, or as long as is comfortable. (Don't allow the mask to dry or pull so much that it becomes irritating.) Finally, wash the mask off with warm water and gently pat the face dry.

Complexion Toner

Toners can be used on both dry and oily complexions. Astringent toners offer oily and problem skins a good alternative to oil-based moisturizers, and they can double as a men's aftershave. Toners that are made with aloe vera or a hydrosol moisturize the skin and also help heal damaged skin cells that cause flaky skin. Diluted vinegar balances pH to enhance the skin's protective acid mantle of either dry or oily skin and relieves the itching and flakiness of dry skin. (I like to use apple cider vinegar because it contains more minerals than refined vinegar, but any type of vinegar will work.) Alcohol, which includes the witch hazel solutions sold in drug stores, is too drying for all but oily or problem complexions. Too much alcohol will cause the skin to compensate by producing even more oil.

Cream or Lotion

Creams are ideal for dry or mature complexions, as they further moisturize the skin and protect it from the environment. For oily skin, use a toner or a light lotion instead of a cream. Just a little oil will encourage the skin to cut down on its own oil production.

Essential Oils for All Skin Types

Cedarwood	Chamomile
Clary sage	Geranium
Jasmine	Lavender
Palmarosa	Patchouli
Rose	Rosemary

*The world is a rose;
smell it and pass it to your friend.*

—PERSIAN PROVERB

dry skin and complexion

A number of essential oils balance skin-oil production, reduce puffiness, and rejuvenate skin by encouraging new cell growth. If your dry skin is also mature skin, use the classic antiaging ingredients: lavender, geranium, neroli, rosemary, and rose.

Essential Oils for Dry Skin

Carrot seed

Chamomile

Clary sage

Frankincense

Lemon verbena

Neroli

Peppermint

Rosemary (especially the verbenone chemotype)

Sandalwood

Vetiver

Ylang-ylang

DRY COMPLEXION CLEANSER

For an added boost, try substituting an infused herb oil of calendula for the vegetable oil in this cleanser. You can either purchase it or make your own—see page 27 for directions.

8 drops sandalwood
4 drops rosemary
2 ounces aloe gel
1 teaspoon glycerin
1 teaspoon vegetable oil

Blend ingredients. Shake well before each use. Apply with cotton pads, then rinse off.

DRY COMPLEXION TONER

To obtain liquid vitamin E oil, prick open a couple of 400 IU vitamin E gel capsules or purchase a bottle of vitamin E liquid at a natural-food store.

6 drops geranium
4 drops sandalwood
1 drop chamomile
1 drop jasmine (expensive, so optional)
800 IU vitamin E oil
2 ounces aloe vera gel
2 ounces orange blossom water (neroli)
1 teaspoon vinegar

Combine ingredients. Shake before using.

oily skin

For oily skin, use essential oils that will normalize overactive sebaceous glands, slowing oil production.

Essential Oils for Oily Skin

Basil	Bergamot
Citruses	Cypress
Eucalyptus	Juniper
Lemongrass	Myrtle
Sage	Tea tree
Ylang-ylang	

TONER FOR OILY SKIN

Without the ylang-ylang, which is too sweet-smelling for most men (and some women!), this makes an excellent aftershave for men.

- **5 drops cedarwood**
- **3 drops lemon**
- **1 drop ylang-ylang**
- **1 tablespoon aloe vera**
- **2 ounces witch hazel**

Combine ingredients. Shake well before using.

OILY-SKIN CLEANSER

If available, you can use an herbal vinegar. I make my own yarrow vinegar for this formula, but a basil or sage vinegar from the grocery store will work, too.

- **1 teaspoon vinegar**
- **1 teaspoon glycerin**
- **6 drops lemon**
- **2 drops cypress**
- **2 drops grapefruit (optional)**
- **2 ounces witch hazel**

Blend ingredients. Shake well before each use. Apply with cotton pads, then rinse off.

problem skin

Problem skin is a complexion that tends toward acne. It generally is also oily skin, but not always. If the person has dry problem skin, you can adjust the facial treatments accordingly by
using essential oils for dry skin. Essential oils for problem skin
are both antiseptic and drying.

Essential Oils for Problem Skin

Basil	Carrot
Chamomile	Clary sage
Eucalyptus	Frankincense
Geranium	Helichrysum
Juniper	Lavender
Lemon	Lemon grass
Myrtle	Neroli
Palmarosa	
Patchouli	
Peppermint	
Rosemary (especially chemotype verbenone)	
Sage	
Sandalwood	
Tea tree	
Thyme (especially chemotype linalol)	

ZIT REMOVER

The lavender in this natural acne solution is antiseptic and anti-inflammatory.

- **¼ cup distilled water**
- **1 teaspoon Epsom salt**
- **4 drops lavender**

Bring water to a boil and pour over the salt. When the salt has dissolved, add the essential oil. Soak a small absorbent cloth in the solution and press this compress onto the pimple. In a minute or two, as it starts to cool, place the cloth back in hot water, then reapply. Repeat several times.

INTENSIVE TREATMENT FOR ACNE

This formula is for those trouble spots you need to take care of—fast!

- **12 drops tea tree**
- **½ teaspoon goldenseal root, powdered**
- **Distilled water**

Combine ingredients, adding water to create a paste. Apply directly onto acne spots. Let it dry and remain on the skin for at least 20 minutes. Rinse.

fungal and viral skin infections

Aromatherapy offers many treatments against fungal and viral infections such as warts, herpes, and the related shingles virus, which causes the skin to break out in blisters along nerve endings. Treat these conditions externally with essential oil that has been diluted in an equal amount of vegetable oil or alcohol. This is highly concentrated, so apply it only directly on the blisters. Excellent antiviral and antifungal oils are tea tree, eucalyptus (especially lemon eucalyptus), lavender, myrrh, and geranium. Use the same essential oils on skin warts, which are caused by another type of virus. (Genital warts need to be treated by a doctor. The virus that causes them is passed between sexual partners, and in women it can lead to cervical dysplasia.)

Many different types of fungal infections appear on the skin, but athlete's foot is the most common. A fungal powder (such as the one that follows) or plain vinegar provide the best base for a remedy to treat fungal infections. Both the powder and vinegar are drying.

Research shows that creams containing capsaicin, a compound found in cayenne, deaden the pain of herpes and shingles. Essential oil of cayenne can be added to a cream or oil base, but be sure to go easy with it, as too much can burn the skin. Small amounts of peppermint can relieve the itching of a fungal infection and sometimes diminish the nerve-tingling pain of herpes and shingles.

Antifungal Essential Oils

Basil	Bergamot
Cinnamon	Clove
Eucalyptus	Geranium
Lemongrass	Melissa
Peppermint	Tea tree
Thyme	

ANTIFUNGAL POWDER

If you prefer a liquid formula, add these same ingredients (without the bentonite clay) to ½ cup apple-cider vinegar. A soft cloth soaked in the solution makes an excellent compress.

12 drops tea tree (or eucalyptus)
6 drops geranium
2 tablespoons bentonite clay

Drop the essential oil into the clay and mix well. Apply to the problem area.

HERPES FORMULA

If applied to herpes as soon as the blisters begin to appear, these oils will often prevent the breakout. Caution: This is a concentrated formula, so be sure to apply no more than a couple of drops at a time.

> **10 drops tea tree (especially chemotype MQV)**
> **8 drops myrrh**
> **6 drops geranium**
> **½ ounce vegetable oil**

Combine ingredients. Apply to only the affected area at least two to three times per day.

WART OIL

Since these essential oils can burn sensitive skin, protect the surrounding skin, if necessary, with a coating of herbal salve, available at natural-food stores.

> **12 drops tea tree**
> **¼ ounce castor oil**
> **800 IU vitamin E oil**

Combine ingredients. Apply two to four times per day with a glass rod or cotton swab to the warts only.

To comfort the braine,
smel to chamomile, eate sage . . .
wash measurably, sleep reasonably,
delight to heare melody
and singing.

RAM'S LITTLE DODOEN,

SEVENTEENTH-CENTURY HERBAL

bathing

Bathing with essential oils is the ultimate aromatherapy treatment for both your skin and your emotions.

FLOATING AROMATIC BATH OIL

The essential and vegetable oils in this formula float on the surface of the water and make your bath smell heavenly. They also make the water feel smooth, almost creamy. When you emerge, the oils lightly cling to your skin, scenting you for hours. For babies, use only a few drops of this bath oil in the basin. Because this formula contains vegetable oil, it can leave a ring of residue around the inside of your bathtub that requires a little extra cleaning. I find the bathing experience is worth it, but you can have an aromatic bathing experience (without quite the same sensation) by adding 2 to 3 drops of the pure essential oils to your bath.

8 to 12 drops essential oil (your choice)
1 ounce vegetable oil

Combine ingredients. Use 1 to 2 teaspoons per bath.

AROMATIC BATH SALTS

Bath salts are another luxurious addition to your bath water, making the water feel silky, removing body oils and perspiration, softening the skin, relaxing the muscles, and soaking away the stresses of the day. For muscular aches and pains, try adding $1/2$ cup Epsom salt to this recipe. All of the salts mentioned in this book can be found at the grocery store.

1 cup sea salt
½ cup borax
½ cup baking soda
½ teaspoon essential oil (your choice)

Mix the salt, borax, and soda together and add the essential oil, mixing well to combine. Use ¼ to ½ cup of the bath salts per bath.

hair care

Whether you have dry, normal, or oily hair, essential oils have something to offer you. In addition to making shampoos and hair rinses, you can brush a couple of drops of essential oil directly through the hair, which holds fragrance even better than skin, so you will remain fragrant for hours.

Essential Oils for All Hair Types

Cedarwood	Chamomile
Clary sage	Geranium
Lavender	Patchouli
Rose	Rosemary

Essential Oils for Dry Hair

Peppermint	Rosewood
Sandalwood	Ylang-ylang

Essential Oils for Oily Hair

Basil	Cypress
Juniper	Lemon
Lemongrass	Sage
Tea tree	

Essential Oils for Dandruff

Geranium	Juniper
Lavender	Patchouli
Rosemary	Sage
Tea tree	Ylang-ylang

Essential Oils to Slow Hair Loss

Basil	Cedarwood
Clary sage	Peppermint
Rosemary	Sage
Ylang-ylang	

HERBAL SHAMPOO

Use a mild and pH-balanced shampoo as the base for this recipe. Baby shampoos, which are generally derived from olive and soy oils, are a good choice.

> **2 ounces strong herb tea (your choice)**
> **2 ounces unscented shampoo**
> **¼ teaspoon essential oil (your choice)**

After straining and cooling the tea, add it to the shampoo base, then add the essential oil. Shake well before using.

HERBAL HAIR RINSE

This rinse is used in place of a hair conditioner. It balances the pH after shampooing, reversing the electrical charge so your hair doesn't have a flyaway look, and removes shampoo residues, leaving hair shiny and soft.

> **3 to 5 drops essential oil (your choice)**
> **1 pint water or herb tea**
> **4 tablespoons vinegar or lemon juice (optional)**

Shake well and pour over the scalp and hair after shampooing. Leave on for several minutes, then rinse.

We can complain because rose bushes have thorns, or rejoice because thorn bushes have roses.

—ABRAHAM LINCOLN

healing the body
with aromatherapy

Most essential oils are germ fighters, but their beneficial properties do not stop there. Many oils are digestive tonics or circulatory stimulants, or even stimulate production of phagocytes—white blood cells that rid the body of disease. Fortunately, many essential oils perform more than one function, so just a dozen oils will tend to a wide range of ailments. It's a good idea to incorporate complementary methods of healing—especially herbs, bodywork, diet, and lifestyle changes—into your healing regime.

When using aromatherapy to treat physical ailments, stick to simple disorders that you would self-diagnose and treat at home anyway, such as a minor sore throat or a bout of indigestion. Think of the remedies in this section as over-the-counter preparations. For more serious problems, be sure to seek the advice of a health professional, preferably one skilled in holistic healing and aromatherapy. Even when treating internal problems, essential oils are usually applied externally after being diluted in a vegetable oil or alcohol base. The tiny molecules in essential oils are easily absorbed through the skin and into the bloodstream, so rubbing an aromatherapy product on the skin will concentrate them where they are needed in underlying tissue. A massage oil blend designed to ease a stomachache, for example, may be rubbed directly over the abdomen; a vapor oil rubbed on the chest will penetrate into the lungs.

hives

Hives—rashlike skin bumps that can drive kids (as well as their parents) crazy with itching—are often a symptom of food allergy. Address the dietary causes of the problem, but the immediate need is to stop the itching. Wash the skin with the following aromatherapy wash. If this does not provide relief, apply the herbal poultice.

HIVES SKIN WASH

If you don't have elderflower to make the tea, use another soothing herb such as calendula. If no herbs are available, you can add the chamomile to plain water.

   2½ cups water
   4 teaspoons elderflower
   12 drops lavender
   3 drops chamomile
   3 tablespoons baking soda

Bring water to a boil and pour it over the elderflower. Steep for 15 minutes, then strain out the herbs. Now add the baking soda and chamomile. Use a soft cloth or skin sponge to apply on irritated skin until itching is alleviated.

HIVES SKIN POULTICE

You may find that even children who normally object to having a treatment smeared on their skin will not mind at all—once they know it stops the itching.

   3 tablespoons bentonite clay
   1 tablespoon slippery-elm-bark powder
   ¼ cup of the hives skin wash (above)

Stir all the ingredients into a paste and wait about five minutes for it to thicken. Apply to irritated skin with your fingers or a tongue depressor. Let dry on skin; leave for at least 45 minutes before washing off.

immune system activity

Some of the same essential oils that are powerful antiseptics also encourage immune system activity and increase the rate of healing. Many such oils fight infection by stimulating the production of white corpuscles, part of the body's immune defense. Still others encourage new cell growth to promote faster healing. These oils work best when used in conjunction with herbal remedies designed to improve the immune system.

One important way to assist your immune system is with a lymphatic massage accompanied by the appropriate essential oils in a massage oil. The lymphatic system moves cellular fluid through the system, cleansing the body to remove waste produced by metabolic functions. Lymph nodes in the throat, groin, and breasts, under the arms, and elsewhere are filtering centers for the blood. A lymphatic massage involves deep strokes that work from the extremities toward the heart, rubbing the oil up the arms and down the neck toward the lymph nodes in the armpits and up the legs to lymph nodes in the groin area. You can do this type of massage on yourself. Lymph massage is beneficial for almost any infection or disease that involves the immune system. However, there is controversy among massage specialists regarding whether lymph massage is appropriate for people with cancer, especially while undergoing chemotherapy.

Essential Oils for General Immunity

Bergamot	Cinnamon
Eucalyptus	Lavender
Lemon	Oregano
Sage	Tea tree
Thyme	

Oils to Stimulate the Lymph System

Bay laurel	Bergamot
Chamomile	Grapefruit
Lavender	Lemon
Myrrh	Pine
Rosemary	Thyme

Oils to Encourage New Cell Growth

Garlic	Geranium
Lavender	Rose
Sandalwood	

IMMUNE AND ANTI-INFECTION BLEND

Use as a general massage oil over areas of the body that tend to develop infection. For example, if you get a lot of chest colds and flu, rub this blend over your chest as a preventive measure or at the first signs of illness.

- **6 drops lavender**
- **6 drops bergamot**
- **3 drops tea tree**
- **2 ounces vegetable oil**

Combine ingredients. Massage over appropriate area.

LYMPH MASSAGE OIL

These are among the best essential oils to address the lymphatic system and use for lymphatic massage.

- **6 drops lemon**
- **6 drops rosemary**
- **6 drops grapefruit**
- **3 drops bay laurel**
- **2 ounces vegetable oil**

Combine ingredients. Massage into the body with deep strokes, especially around an area where there is infection. Consider getting a massage from someone who is skilled in lymphatic massage.

indigestion

The same essential oils that make food tasty help you digest the meals they flavor. Simply inhale the aromas of these herbs (see the following list) and a signal is sent to the brain to begin a chain reaction that can make your stomach start grumbling in anticipation. Digestive fluids are pumped into the digestive tract to help you assimilate the food. (*Note:* There are a few exceptions; for example, smelling the essential oils of dill and fennel may decrease the appetite.)

A massage oil that contains essential oils to aid digestion can relieve problems such as belching, stomach pains, and intestinal gas. Peppermint and ginger ease nausea and motion sickness. Chamomile, fennel, and melissa relax the stomach and soothe burning irritation and inflammation. To overcome nausea, even due to chemotherapy, also try basil. Use cumin to relieve headaches from indigestion, rosemary to improve poor food absorption, lemongrass for nervous indigestion, and peppermint to treat irritable-bowel syndrome. You can also use these same herbs and spices (not the essential oils) in food. For example, sprinkle pepper on your food, serve a peppermint and chamomile tea, or chew on a juniper berry before a meal.

Digestive Aids

Anise	Basil
Chamomile	Cinnamon
Fennel	Ginger
Grapefruit	Juniper
Lavender	Lemongrass
Marjoram	Melissa
Orange	Peppermint
Rose	Rosemary
Thyme	

DIGESTIVE MASSAGE OIL

This all-purpose formula will help improve the appetite and diges-tion while preventing nausea. This is a good treatment for anyone who has trouble swallowing medicine, such as young children. You don't need to know fancy massage techniques; simply rub the oil on the belly.

- **8 drops lemongrass**
- **6 drops ginger**
- **3 drops peppermint**
- **2 drops fennel**
- **2 ounces vegetable oil**

Combine ingredients. Rub into abdomen.

CHILDREN'S BATH FOR INDIGESTION

This bath is perfect for little ones who tend to get upset tummies. The aroma of chamomile is relaxing, and the other two oils will help put them in a good mood!

- **2 drops lemongrass**
- **1 drop grapefruit**
- **1 drop chamomile**

Add directly to bath water. Stir to distribute on the water's surface before your child gets into the tub.

infections

Almost all essential oils are more or less antiseptic, destroying bacteria, fungi, yeast, parasites, and/or viruses. One way to use these essential oils for preventive medicine—even for internal infections—is in your bath. Another method is to rub massage oil that contains them over the afflicted area.

Antibacterial Essential Oils

Basil	Bay laurel
Bergamot	Clove
Eucalyptus	Geranium
Helichrysum	Lavender
Lemon	Lemongrass
Marjoram	Myrrh
Myrtle	Orange
Peppermint	Pine
Sage	Thyme

INFECTION RELIEF

This formula combines antiseptic power for physical relief with soothing scents for emotional relief—the perfect combination!

8 drops tea tree
3 drops lavender
1 ounce vegetable oil

Combine the essential oils with the vegetable oil. Rub the oil over the infected area a few times per day.

ANTI-INFECTION DOUCHE

The yogurt in this formula helps support and reestablish the natural flora of the vagina and keeps the essential oils evenly distributed throughout the water. The vinegar keeps the region acidic to help deter infection. Douching puts the essential oils in direct contact with the yeast or bacteria causing the infection. When you douche, be sure that the bag is no higher than your head to keep the pressure from being too strong. You can add 6 drops (total) of these same essential oils (without the yogurt) to a bath or a sitz bath.

3 drops lavender
3 drops tea tree
3 cups warm water
2 heaping tablespoons plain, unsweetened yogurt (optional)
3 cups water
2 tablespoons vinegar

Combine ingredients in a douche bag. Mix well. Use this douche once a day during an active infection.

menopause

There are several essential oils that help women get through any discomforts they encounter related to menopause, such as hot flashes. Especially advantageous are essential oils that enhance a woman's estrogen, such as clary sage, fennel, and angelica. Geranium and lavender are thought to be hormonal balancers that modify menopause symptoms. One of the easiest ways to use them is in a spray (20 drops essential oil per 2 ounces distilled water, shaken). These oils can also be used as bath, massage, or body oil. (Use angelica oil cautiously; see Materia Medica, page 121.) Menopause symptoms can also include vaginal dryness and loss of elasticity in the tissue, so a formula is provided to help that condition.

Hormone Balancing Essential Oils

Geranium
Lavender
Neroli

Estrogenic Essential Oils

Angelica	Anise
Clary sage	Fennel
Sage	

MENOPAUSE BODY OIL

If this formula is too oily for you, add these same essential oils to four ounces of a commercial body lotion instead of the vegetable oil. The best type to use is an unscented, basic lotion with all-natural ingredients.

> **6 drops lemon**
> **3 drops clary sage**
> **2 drops peppermint (optional)**
> **1 drop angelica**
> **2 drops fennel**
> **2 ounces vegetable oil**

Combine ingredients. Use daily as a body oil.

VAGINAL REJUVENATION OIL

Neroli is an excellent essential oil to use, but if you find it too expensive, this formula can be made without it. The same essential oils can be added to one ounce of a commercial moisturizing cream or lubricant—just stir them in. Choose a product that is made with natural ingredients. To obtain the vitamin E, either get the liquid form or open capsules and empty the contents.

> **6 drops rose geranium**
> **6 drops lavender**
> **2 drops neroli**
> **1500 units vitamin E oil**
> **1 ounce vegetable oil**

Combine ingredients. Apply around and in the vagina as needed.

muscle cramps and pms

Fortunately, essential oils can reduce painful muscle cramping, such as menstrual cramps. The same formula can also be used to take care of most of the problems that accompany PMS (premenstrual syndrome). Research shows some oils lower prostaglandin 2—a hormonal substance that causes muscles to cramp—as well as common PMS symptoms, such as blood-sugar imbalance, headaches, nausea, breast tenderness and cysts, joint pain, water retention, moodiness, irritability, and even alcohol cravings. The best way to use these oils? I suggest adding a few drops to a long, relaxing bath or making a massage oil.

Essential Oils to Relieve Cramps and PMS

Chamomile	Cinnamon
Cloves	Frankincense
Ginger	Lavender
Marjoram	Melissa
Thyme	

CRAMP- AND PMS-RELIEVING OIL

This multipurpose oil can be used for all types of muscle spasms and cramps. Not only is this formula great for rubbing on the abdomen to relieve menstrual cramps, but it's also excellent for massaging onto the lower back to alleviate the aching that sometimes accompanies them.

> **12 drops lavender**
> **6 drops marjoram**
> **4 drops chamomile**
> **4 drops ginger**
> **3 drops Indian frankincense (boswellia)**
> **2 ounces vegetable oil**

Combine ingredients and apply as often as needed over cramping area.

nerve and joint pain

Essential oils of lavender, helichrysum, chamomile, and marjoram are all specific for nerve pain. I know people with serious nervous system problems, such as multiple sclerosis and chronic fatigue syndrome, who find pain relief with the following nerve pain oil. Although it may not offer a cure, it certainly improves quality of life. For carpal tunnel syndrome, rub this oil into the wrists. Use it on the back or hip for a pinched nerve or sciatica, and on shingles (a painful skin eruption related to herpes) to reduce pain.

NERVE PAIN RELIEF OIL

This is a concentrated formula, so rub it over just the painful area, rather than using it as an all-body massage oil.

- **8 drops lavender**
- **5 drops marjoram**
- **3 drops helichrysum (if available)**
- **2 drops chamomile**
- **1 ounce vegetable oil**

Combine ingredients. Apply as needed for relief.

ARTHRITIC PAIN OIL

For arthritis, rheumatism, and similar inflammatory conditions, modify the nerve pain formula (above) by adding birch, which provides the same aroma and pain relief as wintergreen. I also like ginger for its anti-inflammatory properties and rosemary for its deep penetrating action.

- **4 drops birch**
- **4 drops marjoram**
- **3 drops lavender**
- **3 drops rosemary**
- **2 drops ginger**
- **1 ounce vegetable oil**

Combine ingredients. Apply over painful or swollen areas as needed for relief.

sinus and respiratory congestion

About 90 percent of respiratory ailments are caused by viruses. Fortunately, a number of essential oils inhibit viruses, including most of those responsible for flus and colds. Some oils loosen and eliminate lung and sinus congestion, making them excellent remedies not only for cold and flu but also for other lung conditions, such as asthma and hay fever. Peppermint, eucalyptus, and anise reduce coughing and relax muscle spasms around the lungs.

Anyone who has ever sniffed black pepper, eucalyptus, peppermint, or pine knows how simply smelling these essential oils helps clear the sinuses. Cypress will dry up a persistent runny nose. *Caution: cinnamon and thyme are fine in a vapor balm or gargle, but steaming with them can irritate the respiratory tract.*

Antiviral Essential Oils

Bay laurel	Bergamot
Black pepper	Cinnamon
Eucalyptus	Geranium
Melissa	Peppermint
Rosemary	Tea tree
Thyme	

Essential Oils to Relieve Congestion

Angelica	Anise
Basil	Bay laurel
Benzoin	Black pepper
Cypress	Eucalyptus
Frankincense	Ginger
Juniper	Pine
Peppermint	Tea tree
Thyme	

AROMATHERAPY STEAM

Warm, moist steam opens nasal and bronchial passages, making it easier to breathe, and carries the essential oils to sinuses and lungs. Essential oils can be used in a humidifier, or on low heat in a pan of water, to disinfect the air.

3–6 drops essential oils
3 cups water

Bring water to a simmer in a pan. Place a towel over the back of your head and tuck the ends around the pot so the steam is captured inside the improvised "tent." Take deep breaths of the steam for as long as is comfortable, then come out for air. Repeat this several times.

HOMEMADE NASAL INHALER

When steaming is impractical, use a natural nasal inhaler. You can buy one in natural-food stores or make your own with the following formula. The technique described in this formula can be used with any safe essential oil.

5 drops eucalyptus
¼ teaspoon coarse salt

Place the salt in a small vial (glass is best) with a tight-fitting lid and add the eucalyptus oil. The salt will absorb the oil and provide a convenient way of carrying the oil without spilling it. When needed, open the vial and inhale deeply.

VAPOR RUB

Vapor balms that are rubbed on the chest increase circulation and thus warm the body while they fight infection.

12 drops eucalyptus
5 drops peppermint
2 drops thyme
1 ounce olive oil

Combine ingredients in a glass bottle. Shake well to mix oils evenly. Gently massage into chest and throat.

THROAT SPRAY/GARGLE

An aromatherapy throat spray or gargle brings essential oils into direct contact with a sore throat or laryngitis. This versatile formula can be used both ways. At home, you can gargle with it. If you're at work or traveling, you'll find it more convenient to use it as a spray (to avoid spoilage, be sure to clean the spray bottle very well before adding the formula). You can find glycerin at drug and natural-food stores.

3 drops lemon
2 drops thyme
½ cup distilled water
½ teaspoon salt
½ teaspoon glycerin

Combine the essential oils, salt, and glycerin in a lidded glass jar. Shake well to disperse the oils before using. Gargle a small amount throughout the day or pour it into a spray bottle and spray toward the back of the throat.

varicose veins and hemorrhoids

Medical doctors offer patients little hope of recovery except through surgery. I have seen products that contain essential oils reduce the size of blood vessels associated with varicose veins or hemorrhoids (a type of varicose vein) and ease the inflammation and pain they cause. With either condition, be sure to work on ways to improve your circulation with increased exercise, improved diet, and a good herbal program.

Varicose Vein and Hemorrhoid Essential Oils

Carrot seed

Chamomile, German (see Material Medica, page 121, for details on different chamomiles)

Cypress

Frankincense

Helichrysum

Lavender

Myrtle

Palmarosa

VARICOSE VEIN AND HEMORRHOID FORMULA

This formula works very well, and even better if you use St. John's wort–infused herbal oil—which you can buy in a natural-food store or make yourself (see page 27)—as a base instead of the vegetable oil.

- **6 drops cypress**
- **3 drops myrtle**
- **3 drops German chamomile**
- **2 drops frankincense (optional)**
- **1 ounce vegetable oil**

Combine ingredients. Apply externally.

CARROT SEED COMPRESS

When varicose veins become severe, the skin may be ulcerated and broken. If this occurs, apply this compress for relief.

- **4 drops lavender**
- **8 drops carrot seed**
- **½ cup water**

Add essential oil to water. Slosh a soft cloth in the water, wring out, fold, and place over ulcerated veins.

mother and baby care

For pregnant women and young children, use only one-third the amount of the gentlest essential oils required in similar formulas for adults. Be cautious about using essential oils at all during the first trimester of pregnancy; even oils that are generally considered safe may be too stimulating for a woman who is prone to miscarriage.

Massage and aromatherapy can help prevent stretch marks from forming as a pregnant belly expands. Try to apply belly oil at least twice per day. Lavender is one of the gentlest essential oils and excellent for keeping skin supple. It is also a trusted old companion in the birthing room, and many women still appreciate being massaged with this oil during labor to help them relax. In the days following childbirth, add a couple of drops of clary sage to the belly oil to help counter postpartum depression.

Chamomile	Citruses
Frankincense	Geranium
Jasmine	Lavender
Neroli	Rose
Sandalwood	Spearmint
Ylang-ylang	

PREGNANT BELLY OIL

You can rub your own belly—or better yet, get someone to do it for you! Obtain vitamin E by pricking open a few capsules or buying it as a liquid.

½ ounce cocoa butter
4 ounces vegetable oil
25 drops (¼ teaspoon) lavender
5 drops neroli or rose
1600 IU vitamin E

Melt the cocoa butter in the oil in a pan over low heat, then remove from heat. Stir in the essential oils and vitamin E, and bottle the mixture. Massage your belly with the oil at least daily.

diaper rash

Aromatherapy baby oil and powder protect your baby from diaper rash. The oil forms a barrier on the skin to repel moisture; the powder absorbs moisture and prevents chafing. Use one or the other with at least every diaper change. This oil also makes an excellent massage oil for babies. There are several reasons to avoid commercial baby oils and ointments. They are typically made from petroleum-based mineral oil, a good machinery lubricant but questionable for use on skin. Commercial baby powders often contain talc, which may be contaminated with asbestos or other harmful substances. The pure starch alternatives are a better choice. You can purchase these or make your own.

HERBAL BABY OIL
  12 drops lavender
  4 drops chamomile
  4 ounces vegetable oil

Combine ingredients.

FRAGRANT BABY POWDER

Spice or salt shakers with large perforations in the lid make good powder dispensers for this powder.

12 drops lavender
¼ pound cornstarch

Put the cornstarch in a zip-locking plastic bag and drop in the essential oils. Tightly close the bag and toss back and forth to distribute the oil, breaking up any clumps by pressing them with your fingers through the bag. Let stand for at least four days, continuing to break up the clumps. Pour into a shaker and use each time you change a diaper.

Bread feeds the body, indeed,
but flowers feed the soul.

—KORAN

teething

To relieve teething pain, rub the child's gums with a little clove bud essential oil on your finger. This can be hot stuff, so make sure the oil is diluted enough by trying it in your own mouth first.

TEETHING OIL

Clove teething oil has been popular for a long time. However, it can burn the gums. Chamomile is slightly less effective as a pain reliever, but it isn't as hot as the clove.

4 drops chamomile or 1 drop clove bud
1 tablespoon vegetable oil

Combine ingredients. Rub a few drops on painful gums. Repeat every hour or so.

home improvements

Aromatherapy has long been used to keep houses smelling fresh. It can also be used as a natural repellent to keep away pesky insects such as mosquitoes and moths. Not only is it easy to make your own potpourris, room fresheners, and bug repellents, but the ones you make with real essential oils smell better than the synthetics commonly used in commercial products.

scenting a room

You can use fragrance to positively affect the emotional state of everyone in a room or to disinfect the room of airborne bacteria.

Air Fresheners

A popular way to scent a room is a plug-in, which plugs directly into an electrical outlet. There is even a model for your car that plugs into the cigarette lighter! Just be sure you don't purchase one of the popular plug-ins that are scented with synthetic fragrance. Instead, buy one with unscented pads that you scent yourself with natural oil and then insert into the diffuser. An old-fashioned method is to place 3 to 6 drops of an essential oil into a pan of water that is gently steaming on the stove, or into a small amount of water in an electric or candle-heated potpourri cooker. A couple of drops of essential oil can also be placed on a lightbulb ring that rests on top of a bulb and disperses scent when it is turned on.

Modern potpourris owe most of their fragrance to essential oils that are added to attractive dried herbs. They make lovely room fresheners when set around the house.

For a stronger room freshener, use an aromatherapy spray (20 drops essential oil per 2 ounces distilled water, shaken). You can also spray room disinfectant in a sickroom or use it on a kitchen counter. I know one mom who sprays the kids' bedrooms every evening with a soothing chamomile and ylang-ylang mix.

Scented Items

Scented pillows, bed linens, clothes, and stationery offer more ways to keep areas of a room scented. You can scent any cloth, except for silk and delicate fabrics that stain. Use an aromatherapy spray (see above) to disperse the scent where you want. To scent paper products such as stationery, put a few drops of essential oil on a piece of fabric or paper and place it for a couple days in a plastic bag or box along with the items you wish to scent. The fragrance will lightly permeate the contents.

POTPOURRI

Orris root is the traditional preservative used to make the scent of potpourri last for many years. Its light, violet-like scent blends with almost any fragrance, yet it is not overpowering. An essential oil of orris is produced, but it is quite rare and costly, so I use the root instead. However, note that a number of people are allergic to orris. There are several essential oil fixatives suitable for potpourri, including patchouli, sandalwood, benzoin, clary sage, balsam of Peru, balsam of tolu, and vetiver. For the dried plant material, you can use your favorite combination of attractive flowers, leaves, or cones.

1 cup dried plant material
1 tablespoon orris root, finely chopped (optional)
¼ teaspoon essential oil

Place the dried plant material in a closable container, then add the orris root. Using an eyedropper, drop the essential oil onto the orris root, making sure it is dispersed throughout. (If you don't use orris root, then drop the essential oil directly onto the potpourri.) Keep in a closed container for several days—enough time for the scent to permeate the plant material—then transfer into an open display container. This potpourri should stay fragrant for many months. When it gets faint, revive it with a few drops of essential oil. For a potpourri to be simmered on the stovetop, double the quantity of essential oil, using $1/2$ teaspoon per cup.

bug repellent

I won't claim that aromatherapy bug repellents work better than standard drug-store varieties, but they are a good alternative to toxic chemicals. Peppermint is an all-around insect repellent for both indoors and outside. It even repels ants and aphids on your garden plants. You can make a general bug spray with it to keep on hand.

Mosquitoes, ticks, and many other outdoor insect pests hate the smell of pungent essential oils such as citronella; unfortunately, so do quite a few people. The repellent will be more fragrant with the addition of geranium, which itself is a bug repellent. Another way to reduce the insect population outdoors is with a citronella candle that releases the scent as it burns. They are available from most camping and household stores and catalogs, or you can make your own using the following directions.

Natural Mosquito Repellents

Cedarwood	Citronella
Eucalyptus	Geranium
Pennyroyal	

PEPPERMINT BUG SPRAY

In this spray, the soap helps the oil combine with the water.

- ½ teaspoon peppermint oil
- ½ cup water
- 1 tablespoon liquid dish or hand soap

Combine ingredients in a spray bottle and shake before using.

BUG REPELLENT

This repellent will last for at least a year. Be sure not to rub your eyes right after applying it with your fingers; the oils will irritate them.

- ¼ teaspoon citronella
- ¼ teaspoon eucalyptus
- ⅛ teaspoon cedarwood
- ⅛ teaspoon geranium
- 2 ounces carrier oil or alcohol

Combine ingredients.

moth repellent

The traditional way to keep moths out of your woolens is to store them in a cedarwood chest. Camphor chests have long been used in China to protect woolens and silk. In India, patchouli keeps moths out of Oriental carpets—in fact, when Europeans started producing cheaper imitations of these rugs, wary buyers knew they weren't authentic because they didn't smell like patchouli. Modern mothballs are harsh, displeasing imitations of camphor; worse, they are toxic. It is far better to use a pleasant-smelling, natural alternative.

Moth Repellents

Camphor	Cedarwood
Lavender	Patchouli
Sage	Southernwood
Tansy	Wormwood

NATURAL WOOL-MOTH REPELLENT

For more attractive mothballs, tie a small fabric square around each cotton ball.

20 drops cedarwood
8 drops lavender
8 drops patchouli or sage
1 dozen cotton balls

Combine essential oils and place three drops on each cotton ball. Store in a closed container for a couple of days. Place with clothes, using about six balls for an average-size box or suitcase.

flea control

The first time I gave my dog Freckles a flea bath, I expected to see fleas jumping everywhere, but when I examined his fur, they were all dead. You may need to shampoo again in a few days, as this treatment kills fleas but not all the eggs.

Important: If you have a flea infestation, vacuum areas where your pet spends time, then spray the area with a cedarwood repellent.

Go easy when putting any products containing essential oils directly on your pet's fur—especially cats, because they continually lick their coats—and never put them directly on an animal's skin. Instead, use a few drops of flea-repelling essential oils to make a collar (directions follow). The flea collar will help keep ticks away at the same time.

Flea Repellents

Bay laurel

Cedarwood

Eucalyptus

Pennyroyal

Camphor

Citronella

Lemon

FLEA BATH

Compounds in orange oil have been shown by science to be some of the most potent ingredients for killing fleas. Be sure to use pet shampoo for this bath—your critter will thank you!

½ cup unscented pet shampoo
½ teaspoon orange

Combine ingredients. Lather your pet well, because the shampoo acts as a carrier for the essential oil, and the suds help trap the fleas. Fleas have a tendency to migrate toward the head, so be sure to shampoo the face and especially the neck, being careful to keep the shampoo out of your pet's eyes.

CEDARWOOD SPRAY

This spray is very effective for flea-infested carpets, and it smells great, too.

1 cup water
20 drops cedarwood

Mix together and, because essential oils and water do not mix easily, shake well before each spray.

FLEA COLLAR

For the collar material, use a segment of thin, soft, absorbent rope. Make sure the rope segment is long enough to comfortably go around your animal's neck, but not so loose that the animal could get it caught on something.

3 drops citronella
3 drops eucalyptus
3 drops cedarwood

Combine the essential oils. With a dropper, run a thin bead of the combined oils along the rope collar. Let it dry for about 30 minutes and fasten it around your pet's neck. The repellent will last a week or two.

FLEA POWDER

You could use some of the other repellent essential oils for this formula, but I chose cedar because it is less toxic should the animal decide to lick its fur.

20 drops cedarwood
1 cup cornstarch

Add the essential oil to the cornstarch and stir to distribute. Let sit a few days, enough time for the oils to dissipate through the cornstarch. Rub the powder into the animal's fur.

materia medica: common essential oils

ANGELICA *Angelica archangelica*

Magical powers have been attributed to this "root of the Holy Ghost," once a common flavoring and apothecary drug. The oil distilled from the seed is spicy and peppery. The root oil, which is stronger and slightly more expensive than the seed, smells earthier and more herbal. The fragrance of angelica gives depressed people a new outlook on life. Both seed and root oils regulate menstruation and digestion and also stop coughing. However, angelica must be used with care because it can over-stimulate the nervous system. Pregnant women should not use angelica in essential oil form. The root oil also contains the photosensitive agent bergapten, so be careful when using it on the skin. To avoid temporary skin discoloration, do not apply it on areas that will be exposed to sunlight.

ANISE *Pimpinella anisum*

The delightful licorice-like scent and taste of this herb flavors pharmaceuticals, confections, toothpaste, "licorice" candy, and alcoholic beverages such as French anisette and Greek ouzo. Anise reduces muscle spasms, indigestion, and coughing. It is also mildly estrogenic and has aphrodisiac properties. It increases breast milk, balances emotions, induces sleep, and helps overcome nervousness and workaholic stress. Anise is even said to improve the sense of humor and overcome heartache. However, large quantities of the oil may be narcotic, slow down circulation, and cause skin rashes in sensitive people, so use sparingly.

BASIL *Ocimum basilicum*

Distilled from the leaves and flowering tops, this familiar sweet-and-spicy kitchen herb relieves headaches, sinus congestion, temporary loss of the sense of smell, nausea (even from chemotherapy), indigestion, and sore muscles, and helps prevent the outbreak of the herpes and shingles viruses. Basil gently stimulates adrenal gland function, menstruation, childbirth, and production of breast milk. Basil reduces stress, rattled nerves, hysteria, and mental fatigue while increasing confidence, decisiveness, positive thoughts, and awareness of one's surroundings. Large doses can be overstimulating or may stupefy.

BAY LAUREL *Laurus nobilis*

A pungent, spicy aroma is distilled from the leaf and, occasionally, the berry of the bay laurel tree, which stimulates lymph and circulation while relieving sinus and lung congestion. It improves the memory; hence, the ancient Greeks placed bay wreaths on the heads of scholars—and headache sufferers! The priestesses at Delphi sat over burning bay fumes to induce prophetic visions. Some products sold as "bay" oil are actually the spicier bay rum (*Pimenta racemosa*), which is used to scent colognes, soaps, and cosmetics. Unlike bay laurel, bay rum can irritate delicate skin and mucous membranes.

BENZOIN *Styrax benzoin*

The sweet, vanilla-like oil is solvent-extracted (an "absolute"; see glossary) from the tree's gum resin. In India, benzoin is sacred to the Brahma-Shiva-Vishnu triad of deities. Malays use it to fend off evil during rice-harvesting ceremonies. It is antiseptic and antifungal, protects chapped skin, and increases skin elasticity. It is helpful for those who feel anxious, emotionally blocked, lonely, or exhausted, especially after a crisis. Balsam of tolu (*Myroxylon balsamum*) and balsam of peru (*M. balsamum, var. pereirae*) are gum resins with similar aromas and properties. Avoid benzoin oils that have been thinned with ethyl glycol. The thick oil can be thinned instead with a high-proof alcohol.

BERGAMOT *Citrus bergamia*

This fresh, clean scent is cold-pressed from the almost-ripe rind of a small green citrus fruit. Named after Bergamo, Italy, where the oil originated, it scents colognes and flavors Earl Grey tea and some candies. It is also used as a deodorizer. Bergamot aids digestion and reduces inflammation and infection in the urinary tract, mouth, throat, and skin. It kills several viruses—including those responsible for flu, herpes, shingles, and chickenpox—and is a traditional Italian folk medicine used to treat fever and intestinal worms. It helps to counter depression, anxiety, insomnia, and compulsive behavior cycles, including eating disorders. Bergamot contains a photosensitizing bergapten compound, although a bergapten-free essential oil is available. Don't confuse it with common garden bergamot (*Monarda didyma*), also known as bee balm.

BIRCH *Betula lenta*

The bark of this tree is the source of commercial "wintergreen" oil; the chemistry, properties, and fragrance of both oils is the same. Like wintergreen, birch relieves muscular and arthritic pain, softens skin, soothes irritation and psoriasis, and eliminates dandruff. Although people tend to associate birch's scent with medicine or candy, it can be toxic in large amounts, so use it carefully.

CARROT SEED *Daucus carota*

A sharp, pungent fragrance is distilled from wild carrot seeds; the plant is an ancestor of the common carrot. Carrot seed oil stimulates circulation and treats some reproductive system, urinary tract, and digestive disorders. It also enhances skin tone and elasticity and decreases dryness, wrinkles, dermatitis, eczema, rashes, and even certain precancerous skin conditions.

CEDARWOOD *Cedrus* species

This soft, woodsy fragrance scents soap and cologne, serving as an astringent for oily skin and acne and dandruff as well as a soothing treatment for dermatitis, bites, and itching. Cedarwood also helps in cases of respiratory and urinary tract infections. Valued for its positive emotional effects, it is used to increase self-respect, integrity, stability, meditation, and intuition, while relieving stress, aggression, and emotional dependency. Cedarwood repels wool moths and other insects. Moroccan cedarwood (*C. lbani*) is the legendary "cedar of Lebanon" prized by ancient cultures. The pinelike Atlas cedarwood (*C. atlantica*) is from Morocco. Himalayan cedarwood (*C. deodara*) is warm and spicy, and the least toxic cedarwood oil (other cedar oils and junipers can be a little harsh on skin and the body). Avoid all cedarwoods during pregnancy.

CHAMOMILE, GERMAN *Matricaria recutita; M. chamomilla*

A sweet, herbaceous, and applelike aroma is distilled from chamomile's flowers. There are several types of chamomile. This German chamomile is the most versatile and popular, and it also tends to be slightly more expensive. It helps relieve the inflammation of skin rashes, allergies, hemorrhoids, and enlarged veins. It also relieves headaches and sore muscles, tendons, and joints. It treats indigestion, light constipation, PMS, menstrual pain, ulcers, and liver damage. German chamomile is blue, whereas the related Roman chamomile (*Chamaemelum nobile; Anthemis nobilis*) is pale yellow. German chamomile is a more potent anti-inflammatory so is often preferred. The scent of both types of chamomile helps to overcome depression, stress, anxiety, hysteria, insomnia, suppressed anger, and hyperactivity. Also sold as "blue chamomile" are ormensis (*Ormenis multicaulis*), tansy (*Tanacetum anuum*), and wormwood (*Artemisia arborescens*). The last two are potentially toxic, so use them carefully.

CINNAMON *Cinnamomum zeylanicum*

Distilled from the tree's leaf or bark, cinnamon is a sweet, spicy-hot fragrance. The bark is quite hot (it can irritate skin and mucous membranes) and more expensive. Cinnamon reduces menstrual cramps, diarrhea, and urinary tract infections, while increasing sweating and adding heat to liniments. It is an aphrodisiac that relieves tension, steadies nerves, and invigorates the senses. Small amounts spice up Oriental perfume blends. Cassia, or *kuei pi* (*C. cassia*), is an inexpensive substitute from China used in medicine, seasoning, incense, and cola drinks.

CITRONELLA *Citronella nardus*

The sharp lemon scent of this grasslike herb is used extensively in cleaning products because it is less expensive than true lemon. It treats colds, infections, and oily complexions and is considered a physical and emotional purifier. The most popular use of citronella is to ward off insects, especially mosquitoes. It is often used to adulterate expensive lemon verbena and melissa oils, although it is harsher and more camphoric and can irritate the skin.

CLARY SAGE *Salvia sclarea*

Although clary is related to common sage, its action is quite different. It is relaxing and euphoric, enhancing dreams and producing smiles. Distilled from the herb's flowering tops and leaves, clary's winelike scent is an intense blend of sweet, pungent, and heady. In Europe, the herb is used as a sore throat remedy. Clary eases muscle and nervous tension, pain, menstrual cramps, PMS, and menopause problems such as hot flashes, while slightly stimulating the adrenal glands. It also has estrogenic action. Clary helps rejuvenate hair and mature or inflamed skin, and reduces dandruff. It helps in cases of panic, paranoia, mental fatigue, general debility, postpartum depression, and

PMS. Avoid large amounts, which can stupefy. *Note*: Sage (*Salvia officinalis*)—the culinary sage used in cooking—contains the potentially neurotoxic thujone, so use it carefully and not for anyone who is prone to seizures. The small amounts used in cooking are generally not a problem, but essential oils are very concentrated.

CLOVE BUD *Syzygium aromaticum; Eugenia caryophyllata*
The spicy, hot scent is distilled from the immature buds, leaves, or stems of the tree. Europeans, East Indians, and Chinese still use clove bud oil to sweeten their breath and eliminate toothache. It also treats flu, sore muscles, arthritis, colds, and bronchial congestion, and is a heating liniment. The eugenol compound from clove is made into drugs that kill germs and relieve pain. As a stimulant, clove helps overcome nervousness, stress, mental fatigue, and poor memory. Avoid using the leaf, which can irritate skin and mucous membranes.

CYPRESS *Cupressus sempervirens*
Distilled from the needles, twigs, or cones of the tree, this oil's odor is sharp, pungent, pinelike, and spicy. Cypress is found in men's cologne and aftershave. The smoke was inhaled in southern Europe to relieve sinus congestion; the Chinese chewed the small cones to reduce gum inflammation. Cypress helps with circulation problems such as low blood pressure, varicose veins, and hemorrhoids. It alleviates laryngitis, spasmodic coughing,

lung congestion, excessive menstrual flow, urinary tract problems, and cellulite. Used as a deodorant, cypress reduces excessive sweating. It also eases insomnia and grief and increases emotional stamina, helping one to move on after an emotional crisis.

EUCALYPTUS *Eucalyptus globulus*
Distilled from leaves and twigs, this essential oil is pungent, sharp, and somewhat camphoric. Eucalyptus oil (or its component eucalyptol) is used in industrial preparations, aftershaves, colognes, mouthwashes, liniments, and vapor rubs. It treats sinus and throat infection, fever, flu, chickenpox, and herpes. It is excellent on an oily complexion—especially one with acne—as well as boils and insect bites, and for killing head lice. The scent alone increases energy, countering physical debility and emotional imbalance.

FENNEL *Foeniculum vulgare*
Distilled from the herb's seeds, the oil's scent is herbaceous, sweet, and licorice-like. Fennel is helpful in reducing obesity, water retention, urinary tract problems, indigestion, and colic. Its hormonal properties (mostly estrogenic) increase mother's milk and slightly stimulate the adrenal glands. It refines the mature complexion and heals bruises. Stimulating and revitalizing, fennel increases self-motivation and enlivens the personality. Because large amounts can overexcite the nervous system,

use fennel carefully—and not at all for anyone with nervous-system problems or epilepsy.

FIR *Abies alba*
The oil can be distilled from the twigs or needles of several different fir trees, as well as from spruces, pines, and other conifers. Fir soothes muscle and rheumatism pain; increases poor circulation; inhibits bronchial, urinary tract, and skin infections; and lessens asthma and coughing. It enhances the senses both of being grounded and of being elevated, increases intuition, and releases energy and emotional blocks.

FRANKINCENSE *Boswellia carterii*
This small tree grows on the rocky hillsides of Yemen, Oman, and Somalia. When distilled, the oleo gum resin produces a soft balsamic oil. Frankincense treats lung and urinary tract complaints, as well as stomach ulcers, chronic diarrhea, breast cysts, and excessive menstrual flow. Use it on mature skin, acne, fungal infections, boils, hard-to-heal wounds, and scars. For centuries, frankincense has been used to increase spirituality, mental perception, meditation, prayer, and consciousness. It fortifies and soothes the spirit, slows and deepens breathing, and is relaxing. It is said to release past links and subconscious stress. *Note:* Indian frankincense (*Boswellia serrata*) is less expensive and is considered an inferior oil, but studies show it is excellent

for relieving pain and inflammation. It is sold in drug stores as Boswellia cream.

GERANIUM *Pelargonium graveoloens*

The oil is distilled from the leaves of this herb (also known as *rose geranium*); it smells like a combination of rose, citrus, and herb. A light adrenal-gland stimulant and hormonal normalizer, geranium treats PMS, menopause, fluid retention, breast engorgement, and sterility, and helps to regulate blood pressure. A versatile skin treatment, it is an effective treatment for inflammation, infection, eczema, acne, burn injuries, bleeding, shingles, herpes, and ringworm, and sometimes even reduces scars and stretch marks. It is also said to delay wrinkling. Geranium relieves anxiety, depression, discontent, irrational behavior, and stress. It is also used to heal a passive-aggressive nature and to enhance one's perception of time and space. Some aromatherapists describe it as sedative, others consider it stimulating; it is probably an emotional balancer.

GINGER *Zingiber officinale*

Distilled from the rhizome, its fragrance is spicy, warm, and sharp. Ginger treats colds, fevers, appetite loss, nausea, inflammation, and urinary tract and lung infections. Studies show that ginger helps to protect the liver. It is a stimulant and an aphrodisiac, and is used to heat up warming liniments.

GRAPEFRUIT *Citrus x. paradisi*

The oil that is pressed from the peel of this fruit encourages weight loss and healthy gall bladder function. Grapefruit is a favorite with children and is used for those undergoing inner-child psychological work.

HELICHRYSUM *Helichrysum angustifolium*

A pleasant spicy, currylike fragrance is distilled from the flowers of this everlasting, sometimes called *immortelle*. It treats the infection and inflammation of chronic cough, bronchitis, fever, muscle pain, arthritis, phlebitis, and liver problems, and counters allergic reactions such as asthma. Use helichrysum on acne, scar tissue, bruises, couperose or mature skin, and burns to stimulate production of new cells. The scent lifts one from depression, lethargy, and nervous exhaustion, and helps alleviate stress. Some aromatherapists say it helps detoxify from drugs, including nicotine. The French oil is green and is preferred by some aromatherapists; the less-refined Yugoslavian oil has an orange hue.

JASMINE *Jasminum officinale; J. grandiflorum*

An absolute and a concrete (see glossary) are made from the plant's blossoms, whose complex fragrance, floral and sweetly exotic, has earned it a role as the basis of many expensive perfumes. The synthetic version is so harsh it demands a touch of the true oil to soften it. Jasmine is a nervous-system sedative that reduces menstrual cramps and is sometimes used to treat prostate problems. Good for sensitive and mature complexions, jasmine also soothes headaches, insomnia, and depression, dissolving apathy, indifference, and lack of confidence by increasing the sense of self-worth. Jasmine is a well-known aphrodisiac that also increases one's receptivity. The most prized oil comes from France and Italy, although about 80 percent of worldwide production is from Egypt.

JUNIPER *Juniperus communis*

The berries of this North American shrub offer the highest-quality oil, although needles and branches are sometimes used. The pungent, herbaceous, peppery odor is both pinelike and camphoric. Juniper treats arteriosclerosis, rheumatic pain, general debility, varicose veins, hemorrhoids, fluid retention, cellulite, and reproductive, urinary tract, and bronchial infections. It is suitable for treatment of acne, eczema, and oily hair or dandruff. Juniper has been used to provide a feeling of protection and is suggested for those who experience mental or emotional fatigue, insomnia, or anxiety. There is some controversy among herbalists as to whether juniper may overstimulate inflamed kidneys.

LAVENDER *Lavandula angustifolia*

Distilled from the herb's flower buds, this sweetly floral aroma is also herbal, with balsamic undertones. Lavender treats lung, sinus, and vaginal infections (including candida) and relieves muscle pain, headaches, insect bites, cystitis, and other types of inflammation. It is also used for digestive disturbances, including colic, and boosts immunity. A skin-cell regenerator, lavender prevents scarring and stretch marks and has a reputation for slowing formation of wrinkles. It is suitable for all complexion types and is helpful for treating burns, sun damage, wounds, rashes, and skin infections. Specific for central-nervous-system problems, lavender has been used to treat nervousness, exhaustion, insomnia, irritability, and depression. It has even proved useful as an adjunct treatment for some people who have manic depression (bipolar disorder).

LEMON *Citrus limonum*
This distinctive oil, cold-pressed from the fresh peel, is an antioxidant, preservative, and antiseptic, countering both viral and bacterial infections. Lemon helps lower high blood pressure when used in conjunction with other treatments, promotes the drainage of congested lymph glands, is helpful in treating water retention and reducing weight gain, and boosts immunity. Lemon is an effective treatment for oily complexions, bruises, and skin impurities and infections. Like other citruses, it is an antidepressant, increasing general well-being. It also is used to dissipate feelings of impurity or indecisiveness and to stimulate emotional purging. The only caution is that it can be photosensitizing to the skin for some people.

LEMONGRASS *Cymbopogon citratus*

Distilled from the partly dried herb, lemongrass's slightly bitter fragrance is used in cosmetics, deodorants, and soaps (including the classic Ivory brand). It is antiseptic and treats pain resulting from indigestion, rheumatism, nervous-system conditions, and headaches. It also counters oily hair, acne, skin infections, and ringworm. The fragrance is sedating and soothing. Lemongrass is nontoxic, but it does produce a skin reaction in some people who are sensitive to it.

LIME *Citrus aurantifolia*

The fragrance of this citrus fruit is similar to that of lemon, but smoother. Lime is motivating, relieving depression and increasing morale. Unlike other citruses, the peel may be distilled or pressed. Lime can be slightly photosensitizing to some people.

MARJORAM *Origanum marjorana; Marjorana hortensis*

Distilled from leaves of the culinary herb, the aroma is sweet, yet herbal and sharp, hinting of camphor. A sedative, marjoram eases muscle spasms, including tics and menstrual cramps, and relieves headaches (especially migraines), stiff joints, spasmodic coughs, and high blood pressure. It also counters colds, flu, and laryngitis, and it is slightly laxative. Use it on the skin to tend bruises, burns, inflammation, and fungal and bacterial infections. Marjoram helps those who feel emotionally unstable, prone to hysteria, physically debilitated, or irritable—especially if due to outside stimuli. Historically, it's been used to ease loneliness, rejection, or a broken heart. *Note*: Sometimes the much harsher oregano is sold as marjoram.

MELISSA *Melissa officinalis*

Distilled from leaves of lemon balm, melissa's sweet smell is soft and lemony. Not easily distilled, this expensive oil is often adulterated with lemon or citronella. It was the main ingredient in the famous "Carmelite water," a facial toner made by Carmelite nuns in the Middle Ages. Melissa treats indigestion, lung congestion, high blood pressure, menstrual problems, and infertility. It fights inflammation and viral infections such as strep throat, herpes, and chickenpox. Shock, distress, depression, nervousness, and insomnia are helped by its sedative properties.

MYRRH *Commiphora myrrha*

The tree gum is distilled into a warm, resinous, and bittersweet oil. It helps with coughs, digestion, diarrhea, an overactive thyroid, scanty menstrual flow, and immunity. Externally, it treats wounds, gum disease, candida, chapped or aged skin, eczema, bruises, skin infections, varicose veins, and ringworm. Myrrh has been used since antiquity to inspire prayer and meditation and to fortify the spirit.

MYRTLE *Myrtus communis*

Distilled from leaves, twigs, and sometimes flowers, the spicy scent of myrtle is slightly camphoric. Myrtle was the main ingredient in the sixteenth-century complexion treatment called angel's water. It treats lung and respiratory infections, muscle spasms, and hemorrhoids. Myrtle is a treatment for oily complexions, acne, and varicose veins. The scent is used to balance energy.

NEROLI (Orange Blossom) *Citrus aurantium var. amara*

This sweet and intensely heady fragrance is distilled from the blossoms of the bitter orange tree. It treats diarrhea and circulation problems such as hemorrhoids and high blood pressure. It is used on mature and couperose skin to regenerate cells. One of the best aromatic antidepressants, neroli counters emotional shock, mental confusion, nervous strain, anxiety, fear, and lack of confidence. It relieves fatigue and insomnia and helps those who get upset without apparent reason. It also has an age-old reputation as an aphrodisiac. The essential oil produced from the fruit rind of the same tree is potentially photosensitizing to the skin.

ORANGE *Citrus sinensis*

Cold-pressed from the sweet orange peel, the familiar scent is lively. Orange treats flu, colds, congested lymph, irregular heartbeat, and high blood pressure. The sedative fragrance counters depression, hysteria, shock, and nervous tension. Orange is good for oily complexions, although it can be photosensitizing. An inferior oil comes from peel that has been pressed to make orange juice. Tangerine and mandarin (*Citrus reticulata*) are similar, countering insomnia and digestive problems.

PALMAROSA *Cymbopogon martini*

The lemon-rose fragrance of this grass is reminiscent of the richer and more expensive rose geranium, which it is often used to adulterate. The scent varies greatly depending on its source. A cell regenerator, palmarosa balances oil production by any complexion type, but especially with acne or otherwise infected skin. Palmarosa treats stress and nervous exhaustion.

PATCHOULI *Pogostemon cablin*

Distilled from aged, fermented leaves, the aroma is heavy, earthy, and musty. Patchouli reduces appetite, water retention, and exhaustion. A cell rejuvenator and antiseptic, it treats acne, eczema, athlete's foot, cracked or mature skin, dandruff, and various types of inflammation, such as bruises and rashes. Patchouli counters nervousness and is said to release pent-up emotions. It is also considered an aphrodisiac in its native India.

PETITGRAIN *Citrus aurantium*

Now distilled from the fragrant leaves and stems of the bitter orange, this oil originally came from the small, unripe fruit, hence the name, which means "little fruit." Petitgrain's aroma resembles that of neroli (from the flowers of the same species), but it is harsher, sharper, and less expensive. An antidepressant, petitgrain also increases perception and awareness and reestablishes trust and self-confidence.

PEPPER, BLACK *Piper nigrum*

The oil is distilled from the same partly dried, unripe fruit we sprinkle on food. The scent is spicy and sharp. (A more fruity oil is produced from the fresh green fruit.) Pepper treats food poisoning, indigestion, colds, flu, urinary tract infections, congested lungs, fevers, and poor circulation. The fragrance is emotionally stimulating and, some say, aphrodisiac. Though nontoxic and not as hot as ground pepper, it can irritate the skin.

PEPPERMINT *Mentha piperita*

Distilled from leaves of the herb, the aroma is powerful, peppery, fresh, and definitely minty. Peppermint relieves muscle spasms, inflammation, indigestion, nausea, irritable bowel syndrome, and sinus and lung congestion. It also destroys bacteria, viruses, and parasites in the digestive tract. Small amounts stimulate the skin's oil production and relieve itching from ringworm, herpes, scabies, and poison oak and ivy. Peppermint is used in most liniments, although too much can burn the skin. As a stimulant, the scent counters insomnia, shock, mental fogginess, lack of focus, and "stuck" emotions. The aroma of spearmint (*Mentha spicata*) is less peppery and sharper than peppermint, but it is a weaker stimulant. The scent brings back childhood joy and pleasant memories.

PINE *Pinus* species
The sharp fragrance from pine needles is produced from several species, but Scotch pine (*P. sylvestis*) is most popular for cleansing solutions, European bath preparations (it improves poor circulation), and liniments. Pine replaces apathy and anxiety with peacefulness and invigoration. It is sometimes used to help reverse male impotence.

ROSE *Rosa damascena*, *R. gallica*, and other species
This costly oil is distilled, or solvent extracted, from the blossoms. It treats asthma, hay fever, liver problems, nausea, most female disorders, and impotence. A cell rejuvenator, rose soothes and heals all complexion types, and it has a reputation for slowing down the skin's aging. It is also strongly antiseptic and fights infection. Rose is a comforting scent that helps alleviate depression and lack of confidence; it is useful for treating relationship conflicts, envy, and intolerance and is also an aphrodisiac.

ROSEMARY *Rosmarinus officinalis*

This herb's aroma, distilled from the flowering tops or leaves, is herbal, sharp, and camphoric. Possibly the first cologne, it was the main ingredient in the famous "Hungary water," which doubled as a facial toner for dry or mature complexions. Rosemary gently stimulates poor circulation, low blood pressure and energy, the nervous system, the adrenal glands, and the gall bladder. It lowers cholesterol and relieves lung congestion, sore throat, and canker sores. It is used for sore muscles, rheumatism, cellulite, and parasites. Rosemary improves memory, confidence, perception, and creativity, and balances both mind and body. It prevents dizziness, dark thoughts, and nightmares, and helps in the recall of dreams. The smoke was once inhaled to counteract "brain weakness" and to stimulate spiritual awareness. There are several rosemary chemotypes with different properties, such as the verbenone type of rosemary, which is often recommended for use on both dry and problem complexions.

SANDALWOOD *Santalum album*

Distilled from the tree's heartwood or roots, this oil's scent is balsamic, soft, warm, and woody. Once used as a gonorrhea treatment, sandalwood is still used for urinary tract infections. It counters inflammation, hemorrhoids, persistent coughs, nausea, throat problems, and some nerve pain. Suitable for all complexion types, sandalwood is useful on rashes, inflammation, acne, and chapped skin. It also treats depression, anxiety, and insomnia, and helps instill peaceful relaxation, openness, and a sense of grounding.

TEA TREE *Melaleuca alternifolia*
The oil distilled from the leaves of this tree is similar to the closely related eucalyptus. A good immune tonic and a strong antiseptic, tea tree fights lung, urinary tract, vaginal, sinus, mouth, and fungal infections, as well as viral infections such as herpes, shingles, chickenpox, candida, thrush, and influenza. Tea tree also treats diaper rash, acne, wounds, and insect bites, and protects the skin from radiation burns caused by cancer therapy. It is touted as one of the most nonirritating oils, but this varies with the plant species and the individual. It builds emotional strength, especially before an operation or during post-operative shock. "MQV" (*Melaleuca quinquenervia viridiflora*), which has a sweeter fragrance, is considered a stronger antiviral.

THYME *Thymus vulgaris*
The scent, produced by distillation, is herbal, warm, and almost sharp smelling. Thyme is a strong antibacterial for mouth and lung infections, and it destroys intestinal hookworms and roundworms. It relieves indigestion, coughs, and lung congestion and was once a specific treatment for whooping cough. It is also used in heating liniments. Thyme relieves mental

instability, melancholy, and nightmares and prevents memory loss and inefficiency. There are many chemotypes that have specific properties, including the type linalol, which is not a skin irritant like the other thyme oils.

VANILLA *Vanilla planifolia*
The sweet, creamy scent—obtained as a resinoid, absolute, oleoresin, or by extraction using CO_2 (see Glossary)—improves lack of confidence and helps dissolve pent-up anger and frustration. It is consoling, and it has a reputation for unleashing subconscious, hidden sensuality. Some psychoanalysts use it to help bring back their patient's childhood memories. The true oil is expensive; most "vanilla" essential oils and products marketed as vanilla-scented are actually synthetic.

VETIVER *Vetiveria zizanoides*
Distilled from the root, the scent is earthy and heavy. Vetiver eases muscular pain, sprains, and liver congestion and is a circulatory stimulant. Externally it treats acne, wounds, and dry skin. Vetiver is uplifting, relaxing, and comforting, releasing deep fears and tensions. It cools the body and mind of excessive heat. In India and Indonesia, door and window screens called *tatties*, woven from vetiver roots, are sprinkled with water on hot days to scent and cool the house. An inferior oil is distilled from the used screens.

YLANG-YLANG *Cananga odorata*

An intensely sweet, floral fragrance is distilled from these tropical flowers. A sedative, ylang-ylang reduces muscle spasms and lowers blood pressure. As a hair tonic, it balances oil production. The fragrance makes the senses more acute and tempers depression, fear, jealousy, anger, and frustration. It is also an aphrodisiac, although high concentrations may produce headaches.

aromatherapy glossary

Absolute: An absolute is an essential oil that has been extracted with a chemical solvent instead of by steam distillation. The chemical solvent is then removed, leaving a pure essential oil. This process involves no heat, so it is used on plants, such as jasmine, whose fragrance would be destroyed by the high heat of distillation. It is also used to produce a number of expensive essential oils, such as rose. Some absolutes are so solid that they need to be thinned with heat or alcohol to make them liquid enough to mix. Many aromatherapists avoid using absolutes because the solvents are toxic.

Carbon dioxide extraction: CO_2 extraction uses high pressure and low heat to extract essential oils. The fragrance is better preserved than with high-heat methods such as distillation, and CO_2 extraction leaves no solvent residue.

Carrier: Essential oils, to be used safely, almost always require dilution. The base in which they are diluted, usually vegetable oil or alcohol, is called a carrier.

Chemotype: This term is used by aromatherapy chemists to designate a plant that has a slightly different chemistry than others of the same species. These genetic variations are reproduced by cloning or cuttings, rather than by planting seeds. Different growing conditions will often produce a greater abundance of one or another chemotype group. Aromatherapists may seek out one chemotype because it is higher in a particular medicinal constituent.

Concrete: This type of essential oil is produced when a chemical solvent is used to dissolve the essential oils, as well as pigments and waxes, from a plant. When the solvent is removed through evaporation under pressure, it leaves a concrete: a sticky, soft wax that contains the essential oil.

Couperose skin: This sensitive type of skin is reddened and may even show enlarged blood vessels, so it must be treated gently when using skin products or doing a facial. It usually occurs on the face.

Diffuser: This handblown glass apparatus pumps a consistent fine mist of unheated fragrance into the air. It operates on an electric pump—try to find one that operates quietly. Do not use thick oils such as vetiver, sandalwood, vanilla, myrrh, and benzoin in a diffuser unless they are diluted with thinner essential oils or mixed with alcohol—otherwise, they may clog your diffuser. Also, don't let essential oils sit for weeks in a diffuser. If your diffuser does get clogged, or if you just want to get rid of a permeating scent, rubbing alcohol is the best cleanser.

Distillation: A common method of extracting essential oils is by steam distillation. With this method, steam passing through the plant matter lifts the essential oil out of the plant. The oil-laden steam is then forced into an enclosed condensation tube surrounded by a cold-water bath. The cold turns the steam back into water, separating out the essential oil.

Enfleurage: This is probably the oldest method of extracting fragrance from plants. The fragrant part of the plant is placed on thin, warm layers of animal fat, which absorb the oil. Once the fat has been saturated with fragrance, the oil is separated out. Virtually obsolete today, enfleurage was used for plants that are unable to withstand the intense heat of distillation and those whose flowers continue to produce essential oil after they have been picked, such as jasmine or tuberose.

Fixative: Most essential oils slowly deteriorate with age, but fixative oils actually improve as they get older. They are used by perfumers, so the finished product will smell better and last longer. Examples of fixative essential oils are clary sage, patchouli, sandalwood, vetiver, angelica, and most balsams, gums, and oleoresins, such as benzoin, balsam of Peru, balsam of tolu, frankincense, myrrh, and styrax.

Fixed oil: Vegetable oils are called fixed because, unlike the molecules of essential oils, their molecules are too large to escape naturally from the plant. Because they are so large, vegetable oils are not easily absorbed into the skin. Most vegetable oils are extracted by a combination of heat and pressure, although some, such as olive oil, can be cold pressed.

Fragrant or aromatherapy water: These waters are produced by adding essential oils to distilled water, generally ten to twelve drops per ounce. Due to their water content, they are moisturizing and hydrating. They are slightly less effective than hydrosols, in which the essential oils are broken down into finer compounds that absorb into the skin more easily. They are also less expensive and much easier to make at home than hydrosols (see below) as you don't need a distiller to produce them. Spray or splash on a fragrant water after your shower, to cool down on a hot day, or just to freshen your face.

Herbal infusion: This is a fancy name for herb tea. Whenever you take a fragrant herb and steep it in boiling water, the essential oils are extracted into the water. This means that many types of herb tea are valid aromatherapy products. You can also make an herbal oil infusion by chopping dried, fragrant plants and then submerging them in warm vegetable oil to extract their essential oils. (Make sure to stir the air bubbles out of the oil right away, before processing, to avoid spoilage of the plant material from contact with the air.) When the herbs are strained out, you are left with scented vegetable oil.

Hydrosol: The large amount of water used during steam distillation usually picks up some of the essential oil and, along with it, its fragrance. The purpose of distillation is to pull the water out, leaving pure essential oil. The removed water, or hydrosol, can be used in any application for which a water carrier is desired. The most popular uses of hydrosols are as facial sprays and room spritzers. Hydrosols end up containing the most water-soluble or hydrophilic compounds that are not present in distilled essential oils. This is especially true of an essential oil such as rose, which is partly water-soluble. Hydrosols make excellent hydrating moisturizers either by themselves or as an ingredient in aromatherapy products.

Volatile oil: Essential oils are sometimes also called "volatile" oils because they quickly evaporate into the air and dissipate.

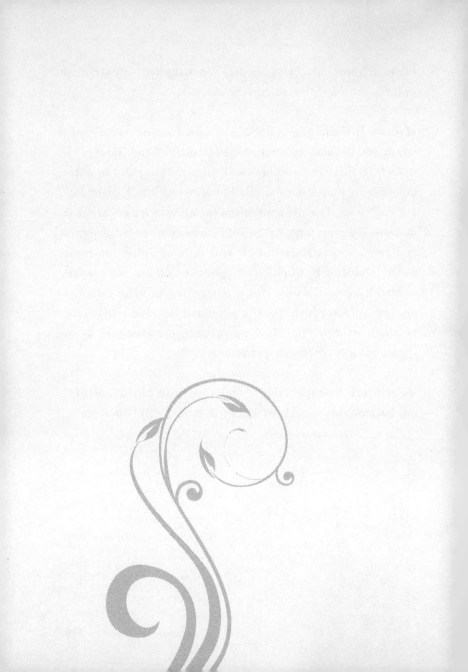

dilutions and doses

Aromatherapy water	5 to 10 drops per 4 ounces of water
Bath	3 to 8 drops in tub
Compress	3 drops in 1 cup of water
Cream or lotion	stir in 3 to 6 drops for every ounce of cream or lotion
Douche	3 to 5 drops in 1 quart of warm water
Facial clay	3 drops in 1 tablespoon prepared clay (water already added)
Foot or hand bath	5 to 10 drops for every quart of water
Gargle or mouthwash	1 to 2 drops per ¼ cup of water
Inhalant	3 to 5 drops per bowl of hot water
Light bulb ring	2 drops on ring
Liniment	15 to 18 drops essential oil for every ounce of carrier oil
Massage/body oil	8 drops essential oil for every ounce of carrier oil
Perfume	one drop for fragrance
Potpourri	½ teaspoon essential oils to 2 cups dried herbs
Room/facial/body spray	20 drops per 2 ounces of water (shake before using)
Salve	stir in 12 to 24 drops per 2 ounces of salve
Sitz bath	5 to 10 drops in basin large enough to sit in
Washes	6 drops per small basin of water

measurements

The following chart will help you through the maze of measurements used in aromatherapy. It will guide you to finding the proper measurements when you convert formulas. Most books indicate formulas by the drop, but some use teaspoons or milliliters instead. The chart will also help you make price comparisons when you buy essential oils from different sources. This can get confusing because they are sold by the ounce, dram, or milliliter. The most common dilution for aromatherapy formulas is a 2-percent dilution, or twelve drops of essential oil per ounce of carrier (vegetable oil, alcohol, or water).

APPROXIMATE MEASUREMENT CONVERSION CHART				
12.5 drops	⅛ tsp.	¹⁄₄₈ oz.	⅙ dram	⅝ ml.
25 drops	¼ tsp.	¹⁄₂₄ oz.	⅓ dram	1¼ ml.
100 drops	1 tsp.	⅙ oz.	1⅓ dram	5 ml.
150 drops	1½ tsp.	¼ oz.	2 drams	7.5 ml.
300 drops	1 tbsp.	½ oz.	4 drams	15 ml.
24 tsp.	8 tbsp.	4 oz.	½ cup	¼ pint
48 tsp.	16 tbsp.	8 oz.	1 cup	½ pint
96 tsp.	32 tbsp.	16 oz.	2 cups	1 pint

resources

EDUCATIONAL SEMINARS AND PRODUCTS

❀ American Herb Association
Kathi Keville
PO Box 2482
Nevada City, CA 95959
530-265-9552
www.ahaherb.com

- Oak Valley Herb Farm Seminars; essential oils; aromatherapy products
- American Herb Association Quarterly Newsletter
- AHA Directory of Mail Order Herbal and Aromatherapy Products
- AHA Directory of Herbal and Aromatherapy Education

❀ The Aromatherapy Course
Kurt Schnaubelt and Monica Hass
Original Swiss Aromatics
PO Box 66
San Rafael, CA 94903
415-479-9120
www.pacificinstituteofaromatherapy.com

- Correspondence course; seminars; essential oils

❋ Aromatherapy Study Course
Jeanne Rose
219 Carl Street
San Francisco, CA 94117
www.jeannerose.net
- Correspondence course; seminars

❋ Aura Cacia
Frontier Natural Products
PO Box 299
Norway, IA 52318
800-669-3275
www.auracacia.com
- Seminars; essential oils; aromatherapy products

❋ Australasian College of Herbal Studies
Dorene Petersen
PO Box 57
Lake Oswego, OR 97034
800-487-8839
www.achs.edu
- Correspondence course; seminars

❋ College of the Botanical Healing Arts
Elizabeth Jones
PO Box 7542
Santa Cruz, CA 95061
800-710-7759
www.cobha.org
- Seminars; essential oils; aromatherapy products

❋ Simpler's Botanical Company

PO Box 2534

Sebastopol, CA 95473

www.simplers.com

- Seminars, essential oils

❋ White Lotus Aromatics

Christopher McMahon

602 S. Alder Street

Port Angeles, WA 98362

www.whitelotusaromatics.com

- Essential oils; highly educational website

ORGANIZATIONS AND PUBLICATIONS

❋ *Aromatherapy Times*

International Federation of Aromatherapists

www.ifaaeoma.org

❋ *Aromatherapy Today*

www.aromatherapytoday.com

❋ CFA newsletter

Canadian Federation of Aromatherapists

www.cfacanada.com

❋ *International Journal of Aromatherapy*

www.elsevier.com

❋ *International Journal of Essential Oil Therapists*
www.ijeot.com

❋ **National Association for Holistic Aromatherapy**
www.naha.org

HERBAL CORRESPONDENCE COURSES

❋ **Foundation of Herbalism**
Christopher Hobbs
541-929-5307
www.foundationsofherbalism.com

❋ **The Science and Art of Herbalism**
Rosemary Gladstar
PO Box 420
East Barre, VT 05649
802-479-9825
www.sagemountain.com

❋ **EastWest School of Herbology**
Michael Tierra
PO Box 275
Ben Lomond, CA 95005
800-717-5010
www.planetherbs.com

books by kathi keville

Aromatherapy for Dummies. New York: IDG, 1999.

Aromatherapy: For Healing the Body and Mind. Lincolnwood, IL: Publications International, 1998.

American Country Living: Ultimate Lifestyle Compendium, with Outlook Book Company Staff. New York: Random House, 1992.

Aromatherapy: A Complete Guide to the Healing Art, with Mindy Green. Berkeley, CA: Crossing Press, 2009.

Aromatherapy: Healing for the Body & Soul. Lincolnwood, IL: Publications International, 1998.

Complete Book of Herbs: Herbs to Enrich Your Garden, Home, and Health. Lincolnwood, IL: Publications International, 1997.

Ginseng. New Canaan, CT: Keats Publications, 1997.

Herbs: A Guide to Growing, Cooking, and Decorating, with Carol Christensen. Lincolnwood, IL: Publications International, 1992.

Herbs: American Country Living. New York: Random House/ Crescent, 1991.

Herbs: An Illustrated Encyclopedia. New York: Barnes & Noble, 1997.

Herbs for Chronic Fatigue. New Canaan, CT: Keats Publications, 1998.

Herbs for Health and Healing. Emmaus, PA: Rodale Press, 1996.

Women's Herbs, Women's Health, with Christopher Hobbs. Summertown, TN: Book Publishing Company/Botanica Press, 2008.

index

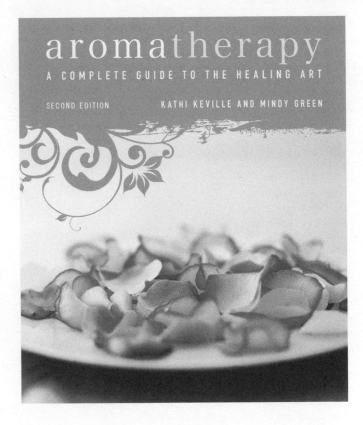